Fit to Ride

Mary Bromiley

Photographs and illustrations by
Penelope Slattery

b

**Blackwell
Science**

© 2000 by
Blackwell Science Ltd
Editorial Offices:
Osney Mead, Oxford OX2 0EL
25 John Street, London WC1N 2BL
23 Ainslie Place, Edinburgh EH3 6AJ
350 Main Street, Malden
  MA 02148 5018, USA
54 University Street, Carlton
  Victoria 3053, Australia
10, rue Casimir Delavigne
  75006 Paris, France

Other Editorial Offices:

Blackwell Wissenschafts-Verlag GmbH
Kurfürstendamm 57
10707 Berlin, Germany

Blackwell Science KK
MG Kodenmacho Building
7–10 Kodenmacho Nihombashi
Chuo-ku, Tokyo 104, Japan

First published 2000

Set in 10/13pt Palatino
by DP Photosetting, Aylesbury, Bucks
Printed and bound in the United Kingdom
by The Alden Press, Oxford and
Northampton

DISTRIBUTORS

Marston Book Services Ltd
PO Box 269
Abingdon
Oxon OX14 4YN
(*Orders:* Tel: 01235 465500
         Fax: 01235 465555)

USA
Blackwell Science, Inc.
Commerce Place
350 Main Street
Malden, MA 02148 5018
(*Orders:* Tel: 800 759 6102
         781 388 8250
         Fax: 781 388 8255)

Canada
Login Brothers Book Company
324 Saulteaux Crescent
Winnipeg, Manitoba R3J 3T2
(*Orders:* Tel: 204 837 2987
         Fax: 204 837 3116)

Australia
Blackwell Science Pty Ltd
54 University Street
Carlton, Victoria 3053
(*Orders:* Tel: 03 9347 0300
         Fax: 03 9347 5001)

A catalogue record for this title is available
from the British Library

ISBN 0-632-04043-2

Library of Congress
Cataloging-in-Publication Data
is available

For further information on
Blackwell Science, visit our website:
www.blackwell-science.com

For Doug Hannum, USA, Three Day Team Therapist. Not only because he has helped me to clarify so many ideas but also because by inviting me to give a clinic at his centre and then getting me snowed up in the great US blizzard of 1966 he gave me the time to start to prepare this book.

My grateful thanks, as always, to my secretary, Sue Langfrey, for not only coping with my hand writing but also for trying to arrange my life in such a way that I could, occasionally, actually have a few hours to write!

Contents

Foreword

Fitness of both horse and rider are essential for anyone wishing to maximise enjoyment of riding and minimise the risk of injury to both themselves and their horse. While most people are aware of the importance of fitness and the problems that can occur if it is lacking, it is often difficult to achieve the desired levels. Lessons tend to be learnt the hard way, through trial and error, mainly because of a lack of appreciation of what is involved, including the influence of important factors such as nutrition.

Without an understanding of the physiology of both horse and rider a work programme will not necessarily achieve the desired results. If as a rider you understand the various factors which have a bearing on fitness it enables you to work out a suitable programme. This should take into account your horse's conformation, temperament, facilities available, personal circumstances, and your eventual aims. Understanding allows you to read warning signs of impending problems, and also the way in which to adjust the programme as you work towards your goals. This is vital, not only to minimising the risk of injury but saving time and money.

Mary Bromiley's knowledge of the anatomy and physiology of horses and humans, together with her experience in dealing with injuries and problems that have resulted from faulty or incorrect conditioning, make her an ideal person to write on the subject. Her knowledge and practical and logical approach to her work makes any book she writes an invaluable reference.

Vicki Latta
Olympic Three Day Medalist
Chef d'Equip to the New Zealand Three Day Team

Chapter 1
Historical Perspective

Thomas Merton stated 'If a writer is so cautious that he never writes anything that can be criticised he will never write anything that can be read, if you want to help other people you have to make up your mind to write things that some men will condemn'. Thus, an opening statement, pertinent to this text 'the majority of riders do not fully comprehend the extensive neural, mental and physical adjustments they must make in order to ride well and most horses lack the preparation necessary to ensure that they are able to perform economically, efficiently and effectively', may irritate some. Others may have a sneaking suspicion that the suggestion may not be far short of the truth.

Mr Thelwell has produced many amusing lampoon type sketches depicting equestrian activities, one of which might have been commissioned to reinforce the reasons that prompted this book. There are two sketches. The first depicts a very fat lady sitting upon and bumping happily along on a very fat horse. The second represents the same pair, and the caption below the second sketch states 'three months later'. Although the lady is still the same shape the horse has become very thin and the expressions on the faces of both have turned from pleasure to perplexity. Exercise has undeniably had an effect: horse and rider are no longer in harmony, the horse has lost condition, and the rider has derived little or no physical benefit from riding.

You do not get fit just by riding. Many riders involved at the highest level of competition, whom, though claiming to be amateurs are really professionals, exhibit totally inadequate levels of physical fitness. Three Day Event riders, breathless, gasp their way through an interview after completing the cross country phase. Recently a senior national hunt jockey staggered into the weighing room where I was on duty and collapsed onto the couch. I speculated that his horse must have fallen out in the country and that he had had to run back across the course. When he was eventually able to speak I asked what had happened. 'I have just ridden a finish', he gasped. He was due to ride in three more races that afternoon.

How can you help a tired horse if you, the rider, are exhausted? How do you prevent your horse getting tired and becoming a possible danger to ride, rather than a safe conveyance?

Riding an unprepared horse is as dangerous as driving a poorly maintained car.

I can almost hear the casual riding thinking, 'nonsense, that only applies to riders competing at the very top, I am not aiming for those heights, I do not need to be fit, my horse is well fed, it gets more than the instructions on the feed bag advise, I have read the handouts, all state the mix will make the horse fit and keep it healthy'. Sadly, a number of my human patients are just such casual riders, injured and visiting me in pain following an unnecessary accident. Many horse patients arrive in pain, injured by lack of preparation, often as a direct result of misunderstanding or lack of knowledge.

Injury figures related to riding in the UK are far from complete. Relatively few studies have been instigated and the Racing Industry is currently the only equestrian body to keep comprehensive records. In the USA a number of studies have been undertaken and the results show clearly the following:

- Riders require education and training
- Riders should be taught control and balance
- Riders should get 'fit' to ride
- Riders should appreciate that all horses are totally unpredictable
- Riders must appreciate that there are no 'safe' horses

Experienced instructors are essential:

- The instructors must be fully aware of the dangers created by inappropriate rider approach
- The instructors should make the rider aware of poorly maintained tack

An ancient Arab proverb states, 'The grave yawns for the horseman'!

When man first met the horse both species were nomadic, both perpetually on the move. They wandered over vast savannah seeking food. Calculations suggest, given unlimited space, that the wild horse walks at least 20 miles every day. Archaeology indicates that from 15 000 BC man kept close to the herds of wild horses, utilising the animals as fresh food on the hoof. Thus man probably walked as far, if not further, than the horses. The first illustrations of men leading horses were discovered in Spain at Canforos de Penaruba. This particular cave art dates from the Mesolithic period, 12 000–3000 BC.

The time period involved for man to realise the degree to which his horizons could be widened if he sat on a horse are unclear. Cave illustrations depicting captive horses between rudimentary shafts appear long before those portraying man astride horses. We cannot be certain when man began to ride, neither is it clear how, when or why man discovered the benefits of improving, by training, the natural capabilities of both himself and his horse.

Historically it is obvious that both man and horse were (physically) compatible when they joined forces. Also from that moment in time the tamed horse solved the problems of over-land transportation for man. Thereafter, like the dog, the first animal to be domesticated, the horse began to accompany man on his adventures and was present at his subsequent discoveries. The journeys made, the hardships endured are incomprehensible in today's environment. It is clearly obvious that both man and horse were exceptionally physically fit.

The passage of time has not negated this fitness requirement, particularly for those involved in competition, as rising standards demand ever increasing athletic prowess, although I fear as the 20th century jets its way through its final decade, the physically active component of the lives of most people and their animals continues to decrease. One example in man is the return of rickets, a condition affecting bone, rarely seen within the United Kingdom since the 1930s. The disease has reappeared, caused not as previously by lack of nourishment but sadly due to lack of exercise, for to build stable bone specific signals are necessary. These signals are only generated during activity. The stresses created by both ground impaction forces and muscle pull trigger the essential messages which ensure that bone will, over a period of time, remodel and adapt, eventually becoming strong enough to withstand the strains created by activity, especially the excessive demands experienced, for example, during competition. Bone adaptation was first described by Wolff (1836–1902), his law stating that 'bone remodels to accommodate to the stresses it experiences.' This feature has also been recognised in the soft tissues: ligament, tendon and muscle. Thus, one of the main reasons for pre-activity preparation is to ensure that all body structures are strong enough to cope with demand.

There are countless, documented, time-honoured methods discussing equine training protocols. Many of these routines are still retained for they achieve obedience and ensure stamina, results having proven their worth down the years. Not until the horse was recognised as a superior athlete and equine sports medicine was born did science begin to examine and address the physiology of the sport horse. Research has now revealed the rationale allied to many of the old fashioned procedures. 'Walk the first mile out, the last mile in' has a sound reason, one to be discussed later in the text. Rider fitness is rarely addressed, which is odd when you consider that the basics for training not only the horse but also the rider were described by Zenophon in his *Art of Horsemanship*, circa 362 BC.

Much of the early training of today's new age horse is still based on these principles documented over 23 centuries ago. If there is a change it is probably word usage, successive writers having utilised more words to say the same things!

Various early Greek translations make it clear that gymnastic exercises for the rider were considered by the riding masters of that period to be of the greatest importance. Not until a prescribed level of physical ability was demonstrated by aspiring equestrians was the riding of a suitably prepared horse contemplated. Plato mentions riding as a part of the education of young Athenian men, but always combined with gymnastic routines. The young Greeks whom he discusses seemed to have been given formal lessons between the ages of 14–18, this possibly because at 18 they were eligible to begin cavalry training. Today, riding has become a leisure pursuit, not a necessity, but it must make sense to prepare yourself to ride before you actually mount a horse, a horse which, in turn, has been prepared to carry the weight of a rider. Then, when riding commences, both horse and rider will continue to condition both physically and mentally.

This book aims to put into perspective and discuss in lay terms the scientific principles that lie behind some of the many training techniques for both species. The knowledge imparted is aimed not only at the beginner, but also at the advanced rider, for to succeed, the responses of horse to rider command, the animal's ability to achieve automatic reactions to subtle leg aids, along with the animal's total inability to suppress, if stimulated, certain reflex reactions, all require explanation. Too often we forget to consider the horse's point of view, endowing the animal with human attributes. Nothing could be further from reality.

Evolution

Archaeological fossil records document numerous equine findings and we can trace the development of the horse from the small *Eohippus* to the modern *Equus*. The interpretation of DNA helps us to plot the advancement of the species. Before considering the implications of horse and rider achieving both a state of fitness and harmonious interaction we must return to the beginning and consider the path of evolution followed by *Homo sapiens* (man) and *Equus* (the horse). Their developmental paths are quite different: man is born only able to do three things, suck, yell and defecate, possessing a brain and nervous system which requires endless training to establish survival skills. This species learns slowly, as do all *predators*, for that is how man, *Homo sapiens*, is described, he is a *predator*. None of the predator species are 'neurologically complete' at birth.

Consider the puppy, the kitten, the fox, the big cats, all are blind at birth, they cannot walk, they are totally helpless. At birth and for varying periods, dependent upon the species, they are completely dependent upon their mothers.

The horse is able to stand, run, feed, see, hear, communicate, recognise its dam, all within 15 minutes of birth. For the horse, to be born 'neurologically complete' is necessary for survival. The horse is classified as a *prey* species. In the natural environment other animals, predators, eat the horse.

In the wild, all the natural horse has to do is to learn herd dominance, then as it grows older, through play, it learns movement patterns which will eventually be required for defence and mating. It is these play skills that we, as riders, harness and perfect, enabling us to execute, for example, many of the dressage movements. These movements are natural to the horse; turning quickly to avoid obstacles necessitates a change of leg to balance; spinning on a circle to chase off a rival is the pirouette; high stepping during mating procedures, the piaffe. Domestication has not altered the animal and the horse still possesses all its naturally endowed reflex responses triggered by external stimuli.

In a natural situation, flight is the first line of defence. Thus, in the horse, both skeleton and muscle are designed in a manner to enable rapid movement. This is made possible by features which ensure economy of effort and energy conservation over short distances. To fight is the second line of defence. Equine predators attack by first running alongside, then by jumping on to the back of their prey to attempt to ground the victim. If grounded, the neck is broken just behind the poll and then the soft belly ripped open.

Reflex, or safety mechanisms, are inbuilt in every species. In the horse, if localised pressure is experienced on each side of the back just forward of the loins, the animal will automatically hollow the back and raise the head. This is a survival reflex that has been evoked in response to the local pressure, 'the message' to get rid of the predator. The effect of hollowing is to first stretch the back muscles, thus allowing the animal to buck as strongly and efficiently as is possible to try to dislodge the predator. Unfortunately, the reflex areas involved are usually (dependent on saddle fit) just below the rider's seat bones. If this is the case, 'boreing down' by the rider is counter productive, achieving at worst a buck or evasion, or an unavoidable hollow outline. Riders should sit *close* NOT overly *deep*. Obviously a badly flocked or poor fitting saddle can cause an animal to buck as it is impossible to stop the natural instincts for survival triggering in. The horses' subconscious reactions will always be 'something is on my back causing pain', so it may hollow then hump, buck and kick until the pain goes away.

Pressure in the area of the poll represents the predator attacking the neck at its most vulnerable life junction. Too tight a browband, causing pressure from the bridle headpiece on these vital survival points, may cause head shaking. Deep in the animal's subconscious a message, 'shake your head or you may die', has been released. Similarly, fighting against the restraint if tied, either for the first time or if frightened, will evoke a terror response. No horse should ever be tied in a manner that does not enable it to break away.

The underside of the belly and area of flank just behind the rib cage are loaded with survival sensors. Why, what does the predator do? It tears open the soft belly. Irritate these sensors, perhaps when grooming, and the horse instinctively twists down and away. If the pressure continues the horse will kick out, first bringing the leg forward rapidly, then out to the side in a manner described as a 'cow' kick. It must be appreciated that none of these reactions necessarily mean bad temper; they are responses to signals, signals that in the wild mean the difference between life and death. The responses are *automatic*.

Man's learning curve is much more complex. He has to learn from being completely helpless to survive. Think of a baby, no concept of danger, no ability to talk, or to balance, or to move. Left to their own devices children learn by trial and error. They also learn by practice, by being hurt, by voice command, by sight, by pain, by taste, by smell, gradually building suitable responses to combat, avoid or cope with varied situations.

Man also possesses reflex responses. Perhaps an easy one to understand is the response of the eyes: dust or grit in the eyes makes them water and there is no way of stopping this response until the grit is washed out. Another example is if you touch something hot with a hand and you withdraw the hand before realising you have done so.

Both man and horse evolve within a female uterus, both begin life with the meeting of two cells, both feed on milk in early life, both could continue as herbivores (consider vegetarianism), both contain a similar number of body systems, but the main differences between biped, *Homo sapiens*, and quadruped, *Equus*, are obvious when we start to consider these two facts.

First, one species, *Equus*, has no need to learn, the other, *Homo sapiens*, cannot survive without learning.

Secondly, that man, a *predator*, has chosen to ride the horse, his *prey*.

The successful way forward is a continuing learning curve, a curve both physical and mental. There can be no instant fix for either you or your horse, and there are no short cuts to achieve total fitness in either species. It is also erroneous to transpose regimes, diets and training methods pertinent to and suitable for man to the horse, imagining they will all work.

Chapter 2
Interlinkage of the Body Systems

Basic concepts

Riding just for pleasure does not, perhaps, require the in-depth preparation necessitated for competition but an understanding of the structure and function of the many systems comprising the whole is essential for all. No matter if they are housed within the body of a competitor or a non-competitor, horse or man, the systems are identical. Thus an informed perception of the factors pertinent to health, termed *condition* in the horse and *athletic fitness* in man, will help riders to understand not only their own requirements and those of the horses they ride but also aid owners, trainers and grooms, even if they are involved with only one horse, to achieve a basis of understanding. This will allow them to make their own informed decisions, rather than indulge in haphazard regimes, confused by what to many must appear a minefield of contradictions.

It is essential to consider *facts* rather than pursue *fantasies* or *fairytales*. *Condition* or *athletic fitness*, however you prefer to term it, may be considered as being 'the state of a body to move efficiently and function economically in response to demand'.

Every sport, every profession has developed a related terminology. Yachtsmen talk of port and starboard rather than left and right and, if listening to experts in conversation, persons untutored in the subject may be forgiven for wondering if those talking are speaking a foreign language. The horse world is no exception. We talk of near, off, cadence, bascule, cantle. To achieve an effective training protocol a basic understanding of certain of the terminology utilised to describe anatomical and physiological function will help, particularly as most modern books, due to the rapid advancement of knowledge, are written utilising basic scientific nomenclature.

Anatomy

The word *anatomy* is accepted as the study and description of body structures.

Most people have a basic understanding of anatomy and every rider has seen diagrams of part, or all, of both an equine and a human skeleton. Many have looked at illustrations indicating the names and location of varying muscles, and everyone understands that muscular activity achieves movement. Most riders have had their horses' blood tested to get an overall picture of health although, curiously, few have a blood test themselves.

Physiology

Physiology is the study of the activity or function of each of the body structures described by anatomy. Before considering gross activity it is necessary to appreciate that there are differences between cellular activity and structural activity.

Cells

Cells are the foundation bricks of every structure. The manner in which thousands of cells group or are joined together determines the type of tissue constructed, and the continued activity of those cells determines the functional activity of each particular tissue.

The activities in which every cell engages (growth, reproduction, absorption, excretion, movement, organisation, irritability, communication, to name but a few) are described collectively as 'cell metabolism'. All metabolic processes involve a pre-determined and balanced interaction of chemicals, electricity and magnetism. There is continual exchange between extracellular (outside the cell) and intracellular (within the cell) components. The components may remain suspended in the extracellular fluid adjacent to cells or stored, to be delivered on command. As one metabolic reaction occurs it triggers another. The second is often destructive as opposed to constructive. For economy, even energy generated by a destructive situation is immediately utilised for further reconstruction.

All cells are continuously active. Amongst their multitudinous features they have the ability to recycle and utilise waste, forming new substances once the original components have fulfilled their purpose. The continual activity and ongoing maintenance is described as a 'steady state'. This state is essential in order to maintain health for all the components of the multi cellular based structures we call 'bodies'. It is sometimes difficult to appreciate that the planet contains multitudes of very important living beings beside ourselves, most with a complex life structure of their own: biologists have described over a million. Also, somewhat surprising to man, is to learn how much we have in common with all other life forms. For example, the genetic code of DNA molecules is the same in all living things: the proteins of plants, animals (of which man is one) and micro-organisms, all contain the same 20 amino acids. When bacteria form lactic acid exactly the same chemical reaction and the same enzyme activity takes place as that occurring in human or equine muscle. Many chemical activities are therefore common to different forms of life.

The basic building blocks of animal cells are derived from proteins, carbohydrates, lipids, nucleic acids and coenzymes, many of which have been metabolised by other living things. Plants, for example, utilise sun energy, photosynthesise and create components required for animal life, namely those which animals are unable to manufacture themselves. Other cellular compounds are manufactured within the body, the availability of the necessary components for manufacture being dependent upon an adequate supply of ingredients acquired from ingested food. Unfortunately, if the supply is reduced or absent, cells often steal from other structures. This is inefficient and leads to weakness. Inadequate nutrition has, therefore, a direct effect upon cells. Because the tissues of all body systems are composed of cells, the tissues will also be affected. All the systems of a body are interdependent for efficient function, so inefficiency in one system naturally leads to impaired overall function.

Structural efficiency

The pursuance of excellence in the athletic context requires structural efficiency and effective, economic usage of energy. All systems can be persuaded to improve their capabilities if they are:

- Exercised carefully
- Fed correctly
- Allowed relaxation periods between periods of excessive demand to enable their tissue to build to meet increased demands.

These factors are a necessary part of the science and art of training.

Before considering individual tissue function the following facts, common to all tissue types in both species should be noted.

- Tissues respond and build as a result of the stresses to which they are subjected during activity.
- Tissues cannot build efficiently if the components they require are unavailable.
- The adaptation of tissues and their response to exercise demands are

directly related, not only to movement during activity, but also to the *surfaces* upon which that activity takes place.

The components required for tissue building by body cells, manufactured by the body, are obtained from:

- the solid foods eaten;
- the liquids drunk;
- the light available;
- and the gas breathed in as air.

All need to be broken down to molecules before they are usable.

The cellular conversion of the ingested products to building components is partly chemical and, as in all chemical interactions, *a precise and correct formula is essential.* Too much of one component or too little or the absence of another results in a poor quality end product.

Neither man nor horse was designed to metabolise chemicals other than those produced naturally by plants and vegetation. Both man and horse may react unfavourably to manufactured chemicals and synthetic products.

Exercise physiology

Compared with anatomy, physiology is a comparatively new science. The early anatomists knew there were bones, muscles and organs but had little comprehension of the integrated working of the body parts. Not until 1889 when La Grange published *The Physiology of Bodily Exercise* was there any comprehension of the effects of exercise. As that concept developed, so, very recently, has sports physiology evolved. Exercise physiology was concerned with the adaptation of the body structures to withstand the active stress created during physical activity and the chronic stresses encountered during physical training. The demands of competition have surpassed any previously envisaged limits and thus sports physiology has become the natural child of exercise physiology.

Equine sports physiology lags slightly behind human sports physiology. Although many of the underlying principles are similar, they are NOT always identical. Man is a biped, the equine a quadruped. The consumed volume and types of food vary between the two species, and the equine has a very poor mechanism for heat loss when compared with man. The lymphatic and nervous systems of the equine are poorly described, even in today's available literature. The equine brain is primarily designed for muscle co-ordination linked to survival, not for skills as is the brain of man. In both species all systems must interact efficiently. Malfunction, non-function or poor function of any one system in either species will have ongoing repercussions, affecting the physical working of the whole and therefore affecting performance.

The systems

Successful performance, at whatever level, depends upon:

- A frame strong enough to withstand the stress of muscle activity (*skeletal system*)
- Well trained muscles (*muscular*)
- Adequate muscle fuel (*digestive, circulatory, respiratory systems*)
- The availability of oxygen (*respiratory and circulatory systems*)
- Efficient delivery of all tissue requirements (*circulatory system*)
- Efficient removal of all toxic waste (*circulatory, lymphatic, respiratory, urinary and digestive systems*)
- A highly efficient and coordinated neuromuscular system (*nervous system*)
- Protection from diseases (*autoimmune system*)

The following are also essential:

- Dust and pollutant free air
- Adequate supplies of fresh, unpolluted water
- Adequate access to sunlight
- A solid food intake containing all the required nutrients in a *balanced configuration*
- Adequate exposure to and experience of all skills required

Fig. 2.1 indicates how the systems of the body are linked.

The skeleton

The skeleton is required to act as a frame built with sufficient strength to withstand the stress of muscular activity and ground impaction forces. Due to survival requirements when considering mass for mass, the skeleton of the equine is, of necessity, composed of strong yet light bones when compared with those of man. The frames of both species are constructed from many individual bones. These bones are arranged in a manner which offers the following, depending upon location:

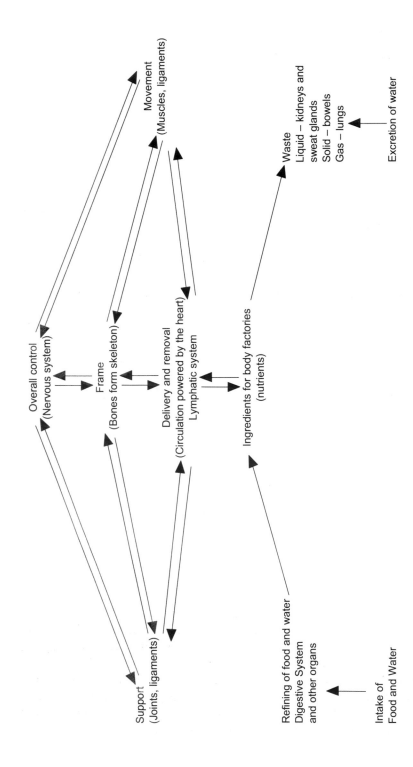

Fig. 2.1 Interlinkage of the body systems.

- Protection
- Protection and suspension
- Movement
- Manufacture

Protection

The *skull* houses the brain.
The *vertebral column* protects the spinal cord (in the equine it also suspends the abdominal contents).
The *thoracic cage*, constructed in man from 12 pairs of ribs, and in the horse from 18 pairs of ribs, houses and protects in both species the lungs, heart, spleen, liver and stomach.
The *pelvis* houses the reproductive organs and bladder.

The bones comprising the main frame are known collectively as the *axial skeleton*.

Movement

In both species the long bones form the limbs and these, acting as levers, move the whole body mass. The bones comprising the leverage components are known collectively as the *appendicular skeleton*.

Manufacture

Long bones manufacture cells, in particular the red cells used for oxygen transportation and also platelets.

Bone

Bone is a living tissue. Throughout life it is continually remodelling and has probably the greatest reparative power of any of the body tissues. These factors necessitate a highly efficient, all embracing blood supply. The strength of bone is dependent upon the arrangement of the materials utilised in its construction, the main ingredient being calcium laid down within a frame composed of collagen. However, as with all structures, no single component can function in isolation, thus a 'mix' is required. In the case of bone, this mix necessitates the presence of calcium, phosphate, calcium carbonate, magnesium and fluoride. *The correct ratio of each component is essential.*

To imagine the construction pattern of bone, visualise a building made from concrete. Steel rods are bent and tied in complex patterns designed to withstand conceived stresses prior to the pouring of the concrete. The steel rods represent the linear arrangement of collagen fibres in bone which are also arranged in complex patterns, enabling the bone to absorb and counteract the stress of ground force impaction and muscle traction. The concrete which is poured into the steel architecture is the 'mix' and as it sets it completes the design shape. In bone the mix is mineral. Bone, just as a bridge or building, must 'give' when subjected to stress. Although exactly the same components are present in all types of bony construction, bone is described as being of two types:

(1) Compact bone
(2) Cancellous bone.

Compact bone, as its name suggests, is very dense; it is usually arranged in concentric rings and forms, in the main, the outer walls of bones. Its texture is much easier to visualise if you look at the cross section of the cut bone at the knuckle end in a leg of lamb. You can see the outer layers of compact bone and an inner central core of differing texture called, in 'lay' parlance, the bone marrow. This is cancellous bone.

Cancellous bone has a sponge-like appearance even when viewed with the naked eye. Lying within the rings of the compact exterior bone, the arrangement of its internal architecture is also patterned to resist the stresses and strains arising from activity. As previously stated, tissues respond and remodel to withstand the stresses to which they are subjected. It is remodelling of bone required in the early stages of training that takes time, for bone is slow to rearrange its internal architecture and lay down an improved internal mix to eventually enable the ongoing stress of impact to be absorbed.

Closely adherent to the outer surface of all bones is a sheath known as the periosteum. This structure supports the mass of blood vessels required to carry nutrients to the constantly remodelling bone and also to collect cells made within the bone mass. The periosteum also aids the attachment of muscles, tendons and ligaments.

It cannot be too strongly stressed that probably the most important factor in the beginning of any training programme, be it with horses or humans, is to appreciate the necessity to allow the bony frame to adapt to training demands. Only by being allowed time will bone eventually become competent to both absorb and counteract the mechanical stresses arising from activity. This process can only occur if stress demands are repeated constantly, but once the necessary adaptations have occurred they will retain their characteristics and the structure is said to have become 'conditioned'. If the demands which caused the adaptive response cease entirely some loss of bone adaptation will, unfortunately, occur. Similarly, if the demands change radically, a new adaptive response will be required.

It is essential to remember that:

- Mechanical activity (exercise) influences bone both in form and in mass
- Bones are able to reconstruct throughout life

These features are required to withstand activity-related stresses arising from joint movement, ground impact and from the traction exerted by muscular activity. Until the bony frame is strong enough to withstand the muscular demands created by activity, there is little or no advantage in increasing those demands. All that will happen is, due to structural or frame weakness, stress-related injuries will occur.

There are many possible reasons for an increased incident of fracture (bone break) in both athletic man and the equine. One of the factors to consider is that we have learned to build muscle too quickly and too efficiently and that we do this before considering if the frame is strong enough to withstand the pull of highly trained muscle masses. To take a stupid example, most people have at some time in their life made a catapult. Visualise the elastic of the catapult as being the muscle, the forked twig the skeleton or frame. If the forked twig is not strong enough to withstand the stresses delivered by the elastic when it is stretched, the twig will break.

Joints and ligaments

A joint occurs anatomically where two or more individual bones meet. Movement occurs at joints as a result of muscle activity. The bones creating individual joints may link together to form a lever which will, in partnership with muscles, achieve movement of the whole, or move one segment of a body upon another segment. Individual joints differ, each having an anatomical architecture suited to its location and movement requirements.

The opposing surfaces of bone ends, in all true joints, are covered with dense fibrous material named *hyaline cartilage*. It is considerably thinner in the equine than in man. The presence of fluid within all joints, called *synovial fluid* (or in lay parlance, joint oil) creates a lubricating mechanism to ensure easy movement between opposing bone ends. To retain this fluid medium, joints are encapsulated, their components enclosed within an all embracing structure called the *synovial capsule* or *capsular ligament*. This structure, in company with the hyaline cartilage manufactures synovial fluid.

To aid joint stability and so that the movement between bones is restricted to that which ensures both mechanical advantage and movement economy, exterior bands of material span the joints. These bands are called *ligaments*. In some joints, for example, the stifle joint (horse) and knee joint (man), there are also internal ligaments designed to enhance joint strength. In both species, in the stifle or knee, these internal ligaments are called the *cruciate ligaments*. In both species, the hip joints also have an internal ligament firmly joining each ball-like head of the femur (thighbone) to the saucer-like craters of the pelvis. Ligaments not only join separate bones together and restrict movement to that which is economic, but also aid in movement because they recoil after being stretched. In the horse some specialist ligaments also ensure mechanical advantage during activity; for example, the check ligaments maintain the position of the important flexor muscles and tendons in the distal or lower limbs.

The muscular system

It is obvious that the body needs to move around, and this movement is achieved by muscle activity. During training, as the bony frame responds to activity and begins to adapt, so the general musculature will also begin to demonstrate improved efficiency. However, it is essential to ensure the skeletal frame has developed sufficiently to withstand the gigantic traction forces exerted by working muscles, before excessive exercise demands are instigated.

There are three types of muscles:

(1) *Smooth* – involved in the construction of organs. This type of muscle is not under voluntary control.
(2) *Cardiac* – a muscle type peculiar to the heart and not under voluntary control despite being similar in construction to skeletal muscle. Heart muscle has its own blood supply and its own nerve supply.
(3) *Skeletal muscle* – generates movement.

Muscle tissue

Individual skeletal muscles are all named. All have an origin, which is the area of bone nearest to the centre of the body where an individual muscle starts or originates. They also all have an insertion, the area furthest from the centre of the body where the muscle again anchors to bone. Each muscle must originate above the joint or joints it influences and insert below the joint or joints it influences. Some muscles work on one joint, others influence several. Each muscle has an equal and opposite partner, for no muscle ever works alone.

Some muscles change texture as they pass towards the area of their insertion. Their bulk reduces and the local fibres compact, so the tissue is renamed and is described as a *tendon*. It thus becomes apparent that all tendons are derived from their own individual or parent muscle. Muscle activity does not occur in isolation. Fuel must also be delivered, wastes removed, appropriate thermal levels maintained, and neurological communication be present.

Nutrients

All nutrients for the body are drawn from four main sources:

(1) Sunlight
(2) Air
(3) Liquids
(4) Solids

Each of these components must be broken down to the required molecular state by an appropriate body system. Only then can the body cells avail themselves of the many essential nutritional components supplied from the complex composition of the four differing sources.

Light

It comes as a surprise to many that sunlight is such an essential ingredient in all life cycles. Vitamin D is manufactured by the body and sunlight is essential for this process. Numerous cell processes require vitamin D to complete many of their metabolic cycles.

The human eye absorbs light beams then focuses them on to a gland called the *pineal gland* sited within the brain. This gland interacts with the pituitary gland which in turn controls specific metabolic activities. Many other metabolic activities also require the presence of light photons. Experiments with brood mares have demonstrated the need for light. Those kept in conditions with restricted access to light do not come into season readily. 'Light starved' people become depressed, and some animal species choose to hibernate during light short seasons, emerging to restart life as the days lengthen. Horses in barns, with no access to the exterior, are denied full spectrum light because glass only allows a proportion of light rays to filter through, and it is the full spectrum of light which is necessary for fully efficient function. Full spectrum light bulbs are now commercially available, and most artists and writers use them to lessen the fatigue associated with long hours at easel or desk.

As we consider the facts relating to health it is worth remembering that today's way of life is very different from that of our great grandparents. They and certainly their horses spent 60–65% of their time in the open air. Nowadays around 93% of our time is spent indoors and horses are also usually kept in rather than allowed to graze in a paddock.

Scientifically documented in the human, the following facts about the effects of light can almost certainly be related to the horse.

Effects of light

- Hormone balance is activated.
- The oxygen supply of the blood is increased.
- The production of the hormone melatonin by the pineal gland is reduced, relieving depression.
- The production of the female hormone oestrogen rises (mares cycle better if they are exposed to light).
- There is an increased production of vitamin D, which reduces the risk of bone breakdown.

Vitamin D also aids the uptake of dietary calcium in the intestine. Calcium absorption is essential for healthy bone, efficient muscle activity and nervous control. While many additives are said to contain vitamin D, there is simply no efficient substitute for that produced naturally by the body.

Air

All cellular processes necessitate the presence of oxygen. The uptake of oxygen occurs in the delicate tissues of the lungs known as alveoli. Blood vessels (capillaries) sited in the walls of these convoluted balloon-like air sacks allow oxygen in the lungs to diffuse into the blood, and carbon dioxide waste from the body to diffuse into the lungs to be expelled. The gases pass across the respiratory membrane, a tissue programmed for one-way interchange.

Unlike man, the horse cannot cough out infected matter from its lungs, making any chest or respiratory infection very serious. In both species lung tissue is extremely fragile and highly sensitive to the presence of inhaled dust particles, fungal spores, moulds and airborne infections (all viral infections are airborne). The airways leading from nostril to lungs in both species are lined with minute hairs known as *cilia*. Their function is to filter polluted air by entrapping foreign materials and irritants in the mucus surrounding them to prevent potentially damaging material reaching the exchange area of the alveoli. If this line of defence fails, due in many cases to overload, particles bypassing the filter area cause irritation, followed by inflammation, this inflammation often leading to secondary infection. Damage of this nature results in destruction of lung tissue. Lung tissue does not remodel to its original, so repair is by scarring. This leads to loss of respiratory area and so loss of efficiency. No doubt the recent asbestos crisis has heightened the awareness of many people to the dangers of the inhalation of irritants.

Equine respiration is further complicated by a bizarre situation in the area of the larynx. The nerves controlling the enlargement and closure of the larynx, necessitated during respiration, are the longest in the body due to what must surely be a design fault. In the equine embryo the heart is found in the area just behind the junction of the head and neck. As the foetus grows the heart migrates down the neck into the chest, but unfortunately the nerves controlling the larynx are hooked around the aorta, the major blood vessel of the heart. As the heart migrates, these nerves are dragged from the area they service down into the chest cavity. This forms a huge loop, for the structure under their command remains sited in the larynx. The length of these nerves, the *recurrent laryngeal nerves*, extends the possibility for damage. When damage occurs it appears that the left nerve is the most usually affected, but no matter which of the two nerves is damaged the horse is left with loss of nerve communication to one half of the larynx, left if the left nerve is affected, right if the right nerve is affected. The condition is termed a *laryngeal hemiplegia* (hemi – half; plegia – paralysis) and the situation leads to considerable loss of air flow. Various operative procedures have been developed to partially rectify the situation and re-establish air flow but all have their limitations. Old fashioned tubing was probably the most successful method – an aperture was made in the trachea and a metal tube inserted, bypassing the larynx to allow air direct access to the lungs.

The air flow in the horse is known as its 'wind'. Horses with respiratory or wind problems are notoriously poor athletes, hardly surprising as reduced oxygen leads to considerable loss of performance.

Man is better served and can increase, by training, the volume of air inhaled, improving his oxygen uptake in response to increased requirement. Man can also cough in a manner which allows expulsion of infected matter but, just like the horse the lung tissue of man is repaired by scarring when it is damaged.

The chest cavity of man is vertical, that of the horse horizontal. In both species the cavity is divided in half by a dome shaped muscular sheet called the *diaphragm*. Man normally uses his diaphragm during respiration in an involuntary manner; as the diaphragm lowers the abdominal contents are pushed down and forward so that the chest cavity enlarges downwards. The lungs expand with the increased chest capacity and air rushes in to maintain a steady pressure state. Man can learn to control his diaphragmatic breathing and so increase his chest capacity at will. Coughing in man is the result of a sudden involuntary diaphragmatic contraction expelling both air and unwanted matter under force. This feature often results in back ache, for a part of the diaphragm is firmly anchored to the backbone and excessive coughing results in stress-related trauma. Man can also move his lateral chest wall to expand the size of the cavity and, under extreme conditions, is able to lift the first rib, increasing the cavity size vertically. The last method is adopted by asthmatics who, particularly during an attack, tend to attempt to breathe with only the upper lobes of their lungs. Unfortunately, many of the positions adopted when riding reduce, or totally inhibit, diaphragmatic breathing, so the rider must learn to improve respiratory function to avoid fatigue. Further complications are now arising due to body protectors, many of which, due to their inflexibility, seriously restrict chest movement.

There is no way to teach a horse to improve respiratory function, a horse prefers to breathe as nature intended which is linked to the way it moves. As the animal lifts its head and neck to allow the forelimb to advance the abdominal contents slide back, pulling the diaphragm, to which some common tissue is attached, backward. The chest size is therefore increased and air rushes in to retain, just as in man, a steady state. As the hindquarters rise to push the animal over the planted forelimb the abdominal contents slide forward, forcing the diaphragm before them and pushing air out of the lungs. You can sometimes hear the horse breathing in what is termed 'rhythm to its stride' at canter (it sounds as though the animal is going 'fuff, fuff, fuff').

The horse, like man, does have other muscles to assist respiration and movements of the chest can easily be observed after the animal has performed some strenuous activity, the horse tries to stand head lowered to achieve an almost straight passage from the exterior to the lungs, thus allowing easy gaseous movement both to and from the lungs. The animals' sides heave in and out and this continues until two things regulate: firstly the oxygen debt is serviced and secondly the body temperature begins to normalise.

FACTS ABOUT THE LUNGS

The horse

If dissected and spread out the lungs of a horse would cover an area equal to a football pitch. At rest the lungs hold approximately 45.46 litres of air. At rest at each breath there is an exchange of approximately 18.24 litres of air. Under stress activity this exchange increases dramatically, the horse moving 54.55 litres of air at each breath. In the ridden horse during activity lung function is somewhat restricted, principally by the girths but also to a degree by rider weight. Try to run up a hill with a tight belt at nipple level, carrying a heavy knapsack on your back, and you will appreciate restrictions similar to that which the horse enjoys.

Man

A human's lungs dissected and spread out would cover an area equal to a tennis court. At rest the lungs contain approximately 2.52 litres of air. At rest at each breath there is an exchange of approximately 0.35 litres of air. Just as with the horse, under stress activity there is the capacity, in a healthy athlete, to raise the volume of air to 6.0 litres, exchanging 4.5 litres at each full breath (inspiration and expiration).

Liquids

Adequate water is an essential for life. Fluid loss and depletion of liquids from the body results in a condition termed dehydration. This state not only reduces performance but may even cause death.

The balance of the distribution of liquids throughout all body systems is regulated by *electrolytes*. These are ions derived from differing minerals and are capable of carrying an electrical charge. Those transporting a *negative* charge are known as *anions*, those transporting a *positive* charge are termed *cations*. The presence of these ions, in the correct balance, is essential not only for liquid balance, muscle activity and nerve transmission, but also for the maintenance of the proper structure and function of all the tissues and organs in both horse and man.

The principal electrolytes are:

Na	Sodium	cation	extracellular
K	Potassium	cation	intracellular
Cl	Chloride	anion	extracellular
Ca_2	Calcium	cation	
Mg_2	Magnesium	cation	

The body cannot store electrolytes against need. Cell function is disturbed if electrolytes are not in balance. Unless excessive sweating occurs neither species lose enough electrolytes to necessitate replenishment as there are sufficient electrolytes already present in food for any normal deficiency to be rectified. Supplementation should only be necessary if *excessive* sweating has occurred because electrolytes are lost in sweat. Should supplementation be needed electrolytes are best administered in a liquid form because their ability to pass from the intestines into the body is dependent upon their being suspended in liquid. If fed as dry matter some of the intestinal liquids will be recruited for their suspension and, at worse, if that liquid is inadequate, fluid from intracellular sources will be utilised, upsetting the 'steady state' in the robbed area.

Minerals and vitamins can also be 'water fed' provided they do not taint or change the taste of the drinking water radically. Water sweetened by a very small amount of molasses will often tempt bad drinkers. Many competitors travel with 'home water' to events to ensure their horses will not refuse to drink. Stream or spring water always kept horses healthy but, unless you live in an area where agrochemicals are a rarity rather than the norm, the water supply will now be heavily contaminated, particularly with nitrates. There are levels of toxicity published; acceptable toxic levels vary from nation to nation but the UK allows rather higher levels than do most other countries. Many people now drink bottled water rather than tap water, poor horses. It is perfectly acceptable to ask the local water authority for a chemical analysis of the water in an area, and it is common knowledge that the water quality throughout the UK is being investigated by the EU Commission. New legislation, determining acceptable levels of chemicals, will be enforced in 1999.

The high levels of nitrates must be a cause, amid other factors, for concern. The nitrate concern arises due to the indisputable proven fact that, in the presence of excess nitrates, blood haemoglobin can be converted from the ferrous to the ferric state. If this occurs haemoglobin can no longer combine with, and therefore transport, oxygen. The EEC has set a recommended maximum of 25 mg/l with an absolute maximum of 50 mg/l for water borne nitrates. As oxygen is essential for performance and health it is easy to speculate that contaminated water can reduce general health, overall performance and fitness levels.

Solid foods

Despite all the advice and the endless books there is little real understanding regarding nutritional requirements in the horse. Even in man, new, supposedly more effective methods of eating are continually being suggested. The horse has developed a digestive system efficient for the conversion of naturally growing herbs and grasses and the animals evolved in areas of beneficial herbage, secondary to soil conditions and mineral availability. Man learned by experiment those plants most suited to his needs as he followed his 'meat on the hoof'.

Both species start the breakdown of solid matter by grinding or pulverising their food, and this is the function of the teeth. Both species have a cross chew action, but the horse evolved a longer jaw to pulverise woody material.

If, and only if, food has been broken down efficiently in the mouth can the stomach initiate the second part of the complex series of food break-down which we call *digestion*. Following digestion, the food is *absorbed* in the gut. The horse is most efficient at extracting nutrients when fed little and often and domestication has not changed this. The wild horse walks up to 20 miles a day to find all its requirements, grazing as it goes, and this continual movement enhances gut motility (known as *peristalsis*) thus improving nutrient uptake. Man too is meant to be on the move for, just like the horse, the intestines benefit from movement to complement the process of digestion. Elderly people who sit in rocking chairs, as their life becomes more sedentary, have a better health record when compared with totally 'static' contemporaries! Early men were leaner than modern man and, undoubtedly today both man and horse are grossly over-fed, over-supplemented and overweight, straining all the body systems.

Delivery and removal

Circulation

The circulatory system refers to blood flow, a complex, all embracing, closed circuit system powered by the heart and divided for ease of description into three.

- *Arterial*, responsible for delivery
- *Capillary* network, for interchange both into and out of the tissues.
- *Venous*, responsible for waste removal.

To consider this system as a separate entity is a great mistake, but unfortunately it is unavoidable descriptively, it should be possible to describe the respiratory and circulatory systems as a single unit but that is not the manner adopted by anatomists or physiologists, despite the fact that the body cannot survive without oxygen any more than it can survive without a heart, because the heart is needed to power arterial blood flow.

The body can survive for long periods without movement or food, but not for long without liquid. Blood should be considered as a 'porter' liquid, moving a variety of components around the body suspended within its own liquid medium, the plasma, or attached, as in the case of oxygen molecules, to specialist 'trolley' cells.

The invasion of all body tissues by a complex network of capillaries, the minute blood bearing tubules with walls the thickness of a single cell, is almost impossible to comprehend. When we consider that every single muscle fibre requires delivery and removal facilities, and also that when you consider individual muscle fibres range in diameter from 80 µm (micro metres) down to 10 µm, and that several thousand fibres are needed to complete a single muscle, the complexity of the system begins to become apparent. Capillaries derive their useful components from the arterial vessels communicating between all the differing systems, these vessels having in turn collected the usable goods from other capillary networks.

All systems of the body are well endowed with arteries, capillaries and veins. The system in the capillaries is two way. Waste moves by diffusing into the capillaries, usable components diffuse out to body cells as required. Waste-laden blood moves through the capillary network then slowly into the veins and onward to the waste disposal centres. At these centres the waste is sifted and any useful components are recycled. Non-reusable components are excreted – gas from the lungs, liquids as urine, solids as faeces.

The heart is the muscular pump responsible for forcing arterial blood through the primary section of the delivery network of large arteries. The heart is a specialised muscle and, like the skeletal and muscular systems, needs to be prepared for exercise activity.

Waste disposal

Solids

Every process involved in conversion of a substance from one state to another generates waste; if you light a fire, you enjoy the heat, but you are left with ash, a residue, often mineral rich which should be put back into the soil. The metabolic processes of the body are no different. Equine faeces (droppings) are solid based but still contain nutrients which were not required by the body. Man's faeces are the same and are used in many so called 'under developed countries' as a fertiliser named 'night soil'.

The condition of the faeces in both man and horse can be used as a health indicator.

The faeces of a horse should have the following features:

- They should be 'formed'
- They should not be too liquid
- They should not be dry, solid or pellet-like
- There should be no obnoxious or sour smell
- They should not contain undigested matter, for example whole oats.

The droppings of each horse will differ, but any change from normal should be noted and, if possible, a reason sought – change of food, new hay, not drinking enough?

Liquids

Urine, like faeces, contains components which are not required by the body. After filtering in the kidneys, where reusable compounds are extracted (particularly calcium) the urine passes to the bladder to be stored prior to excretion. Excreted urine in both man and horse:

- Should be clear
- Should be plentiful, not scant
- Should be passed easily
- Should have no smell
- Should not be thick, deep yellow or pus coloured.

The condition of urine in both species is both a health and hydration indicator.

Gaseous waste

Waste gases are excreted, in the main, from the lungs, thus the lungs are concerned with respiratory waste. Excess gas produced within the intestines and passed as 'wind' is an indicator of digestive disturbance.

Sweat

Sweating acts both as a method of temperature reduction and the excretion of waste. In certain circumstances sweating can result in disastrous loss of liquid and electrolytes.

Resistance and recovery

The body has many fail safety mechanisms in-built and not under conscious control. Grit in the eye recruits the production, by the tear glands, of extra liquid to flush out the dirt. The immune system of the body has in-built planned resistance. The main system designed to deal with any invasion is the *lymphatic system*. The lymphatic system can produce protective cells to fight any invasion, and specialist cells to mop up, or ingest, any by-products resulting from an invasion.

Exposure to disease-causing organisms in small doses ensures that resistance programmes are created then stored in the body. Programmes can also be initiated by the injecting of a minute amount of specialist chemical messengers to initiate the planning and storage of a suitable resistance programme.

Unfortunately, viruses do not behave in the same way as bacteria. This is why the ability of the virus to change the goal posts make it so difficult to either protect against viral invasion, or to combat the effects if they do invade.

Nervous system

For simplicity, the nervous system will be divided into:

- Central nervous system (the brain and spinal cord)
- Peripheral nervous system (motor control)

In addition, the nerves may be divided into *autonomic* or *involuntary* nerves (those not under conscious control) and the *voluntary* nerves (those under conscious control).

Central nervous system

The central nervous system comprises the brain and its extension (the spinal cord), a cord passing from the base of the brain (brain stem) into the body mass and protected within the vertebral column. The brain acts as a highly complex computer, analysing all incoming information, deciding upon the appropriate responses, and dispatching signals to achieve the responses required. These signals are multi-delivery as more than one tissue and system is usually involved.

The spinal cord, if seen magnified and in cross section, would resemble a main telephone cable. Multitudinous bundles of fibres are arranged in tracts, each tract having its own specific communication function. All commands from the brain to all the body parts, and the responses from all body parts to the brain, travel along one of the many tracts within the spinal cord. Damage to any part of the central nervous system is not really pertinent to a text on improving athletic ability but athletes do occasionally sustain injuries to their central nervous system. The tissues of this system *never recover* from serious injury, thus an accident which destroys central nervous tissue will, dependent upon the area in which the injury is sustained, render that area incapable of ever again transmitting or receiving signals. If man or horse severs their spinal cord they become paralysed and all function beyond the level of damage is lost. A horse with damage to its spinal cord is termed a 'wobbler', whereas man becomes either a paraplegic or, if the lesion is high in the neck, a quadraplegic. If trauma occurs within the main brain all functional commands cease from the area of damage.

Peripheral nervous system

The peripheral nervous system describes nerves found within the body mass. These nerves originate from the spinal cord and are given off in pairs, one to the right and one to the left of the body, emerging through gaps formed between the individual vertebral bodies. These gaps are created by both the presence of the intravertebral disc and bone design. Motor nerves deliver messages of command, while sensory nerves report back to the brain.

The commands to muscles are chemically induced through the ends of fibres from the controlling nerve. Training the nervous system in man is a necessity for survival, but in the horse survival skills are already inherent or imprinted. Man has to learn how to integrate with the equine system and so achieve the interaction necessary to utilise the hereditary abilities of the horse. This is the only way to achieve success.

Autonomic nervous system

This system communicates with the heart, lungs, digestive system and all other systems not under voluntary control.

This section has aimed to give a brief outline of the interlinkage of the body systems, because planning a fitness programme, be it for competition or just for pleasure, does necessitate some knowledge of the complex functions of the body, in order to appreciate the part that exercise and diet play in influencing the whole body.

Chapter 3
Preparation Explained

The skills: harnessing reflexes

The first and most important factor for any rider, trainer or groom to appreciate is the significance and meaning of the term 'reflex response'. There are two basic categories of reflex action. Firstly, those already pre-programmed into the brain, designed primarily for body preservation and defence, secondly those which can, with careful training, become a habitual response to a specific signal.

Consider the first type, those pre-programmed or already present in both species. The inhalation of dust or foreign particles is potentially harmful to lung tissue and thus to oxygen uptake. In man's body, the self defence mechanism, designed to combat this potentially dangerous situation, is a sneeze. You do not have to learn how to sneeze, a sneeze occurs without any conscious thought as an immediate involuntary response evoked by a given stimulus. Other programmed reflexes include waste elimination, for example, when the bladder is full the need to urinate is triggered. The pupil of the eye responds automatically without conscious control to the strength or weakness of available light, there is an automatic adjustment of balance for control of posture, for coordination of movement, for temperature control, heart rate, respiratory rate and depth. In fact, the functions of the body necessary for life occur without conscious effort, they are all *reflex*. In many instances one reflex action triggers a series of responses, creating a 'chain reaction'. Most activities are a series of events, rather than a single action. If for some reason the complex chain of reactions is broken, interfered with, or does not 'trigger in', the particular activity cannot occur.

An equine example of a chain breakdown is demonstrable by considering the numerous coordinated movements and muscular activities required to enable a horse to get up after it has been lying down. The horse must first bend or flex its neck to one side. This is the only movement that can activate the chain reaction which enables the animal to get up. If the head is held down, preventing the very first movement required to activate the full chain, the animal is unable to instigate the series of interactions needed to achieve a standing posture. Thus, sitting on a horse's head will keep it on the ground, the time honoured method of making a horse remain recumbent after injury or accident when it is struggling to rise. The trick is described in detail in all early writings concerning horse husbandry. Those who adopted this method of restraint at the beginning of the horse/man relationship had no idea they were breaking a complex reflex pattern or, described in a physiological manner, that they were inhibiting a series of neurological reactions. They just knew that it worked, a very good example of a proven practical method now scientifically explained.

Pre-programmed reflex responses are stored in the brains of all species. Some, very primitive at birth, are refined progressively, others can be utilised and adapted to improve skills and performance. The art of training the horse and the art of riding require both man and horse to master new skills and to store the coordination of movements required for each new skill in the brain. This can only be achieved by repeating the movement combinations required again and again, always using the same signal, until the desired movement reaction occurs immediately, in response to the given signal, without conscious thought. The response to the signal has become automatic, and a new 'reflex reaction' has been established. The ability to evoke these automatic responses in the horse when it is ridden can only be achieved successfully if the rider gives exactly the same command as that utilised when teaching the skill or movement. If rider commands differ, the horse will become confused. Rider signals or commands are known in equestrianism as 'aids'. The rider first needs to learn to 'feel' through seat, thighs and hands while adopting a posture totally foreign to man and to master a series of balanced, bilateral movements.

The skill of the horse is to respond to the aids, the skill of the rider is to learn to give the correct aids.

Touch (neural input) in the horse

The horse responds naturally to pressure in certain areas of its body. One of the arts of training is to educate and coordinate these areas of sensitivity, thereby eventually achieving immediate responses to almost invisible commands. This indicates that the fine tuning of reflexes has been established.

The touch method of communication between horse and rider was explored and documented by the early schools of riding in Europe, the commands becoming known as the *aids* and the training as *dressage*. Unfortunately, instead of explaining this basic training required to enable the horse to become a safe, responsible conveyance, whatever its eventual lifestyle, the teachers and books on riding tend to require far too much of the novice rider (this attitude might be compared to trying to teach a child the theory of relativity before it has mastered its ABC).

The horse, contrary to some beliefs, has a remarkably retentive memory and, provided it is not confused, learns to respond to given signals very quickly. The Masters of the European Schools taught that communication via touch was two-way, the horse responding to rider touch and the rider learning to respond to signals delivered by the movements of the horse. To ride a well balanced horse, one that imparts a sensation of lifting beneath you and moves as though on springs, is an unforgettable experience. To those who have never had the luck to feel this, try to find and sit in a Citroen car, the model that lifts before you drive off. This experience gives some idea of what it feels like if a horse lifts under you. The horse will impart signals, via the *reins* to your *hands*, through its *back* to your *buttocks*, and via *your legs* to the movements of *its legs*. The relationship between rider and horse is essential but it takes a long time to learn.

Touch (neural input) in the rider

Other than voice the rider has three methods of communication with the horse:

- Via the sensitivity of hands
- Via the sensitivity and slight pushing action of the muscles of rider buttocks
- Via the compression of the lower leg against the sides of the horse

We have just said that the horse will communicate to the rider, and that the rider should experience this through hands, buttocks and legs, and that these methods of communication, when man commands the horse from these three areas, are known as *aids*. Perhaps a good way to envisage aids is to consider Semaphore or the Morse Code. Both utilise a combination of recognised signals to send comprehensive messages from one party to another in situations where command by voice is inappropriate or, due to distance, impossible. If the signaller does not signal correctly, the message will be incomprehensible and the response incorrect or absent. This is exactly what will happen if signals from rider to horse are not as clear as they should be; the messages must be given clearly and must mirror those to which the horse learned to respond during early training. If the signals received are not understood by the horse, the animal will either fail to respond, or respond incorrectly.

It is very important for the rider to learn communication skills and they are best learned on a *school master*, that is, a well trained horse who will only respond to the appropriate, correctly delivered signals. The *aids* are logical, they are a language and, just as one learns a new spoken language, so the rider must first learn the basic aids, then practise this new language. As basic communication skills improve, so those of a more complex nature can be learned and attempted. Remember, practise makes perfect, but Rome was not built in a day.

Considerations for the development of riding skills in man

As we have said earlier humans are classified as predators. Unlike prey species, predators are not neurologically complete at birth: they are born helpless. Although the human race considers it is superior to all other species, this is not apparent at birth! The educational curve of all predators is one of slow learning necessitating a great deal of experimentation. This curve is applicable to the new rider.

After endless repetitions, the brain records the required response to a stimulus or position, and the action can then occur without conscious thought. A child learning to tie a shoelace is a simple example. Every coordination, every activity must be explored and learned: the baby must learn to focus, to coordinate its movements enabling it to grasp, to move, to crawl, to sit, to balance, to stand, to talk. Young predators have no instinctive appreciation of danger. For example, until a child feels pain as the result of an experience, it will continue, unwittingly, to endanger itself. As comprehension improves, along with the ability to think for itself, so the young predator will learn to consider before it acts. Self preservation, self defence and self control are all acquired skills. Aboriginal man, even though also helpless at birth, but living in a natural environment, develops a far higher standard of natural skills than his 'civilised' contemporaries. His sense of smell is very subtle, his hearing acute, his observation continual. Rhythm of movement and balance mirror that of a highly trained gymnast, his body is mobile and, unless subjected to inadequate nutrition or imposed illness from outside sources, he is very healthy, often living well into the hundreds while still leading an active life. Tiresomely, civilisation has subdued many of our useful natural aptitudes.

Riding is a learning curve and learning to perfect it is an art form. Riding is not just a skill, interaction with another species is an art. Notable people have developed this ability and in modern parlance are tabled as communicators. In today's world Linda Tellington-Jones and Monty

Roberts are two who immediately spring to mind, but there are many others who remain unrecognised. Those who wish to be horsemen, as opposed to those who just wish to sit on a horse, using the animal as a means of conveyance, must attempt to rediscover, redevelop and retrain hidden, naturally occurring abilities. Only by doing this is it possible to achieve the body and mind coordination necessary and unique to riding. No other sport, no other occupation, demands such a complexity of muscle activity, joint repositioning, continual shifts of balance and the ability to work the body, positioned as it is in a manner totally unrelated to any previously learned coordination patterns. None of the positions required when riding have been previously learned because, as the baby progressed from lying to sitting, to crawling, to being balanced in the vertical, all coordination has been based on diagonal movement patterns adopted by bipeds.

Riding demands that both sides of the rider's body work in unison as a perfectly matched pair, at trot both of the rider's knees must move together. This is contrary to moving over ground at walk or run when one knee is straight, the other bent. Other than those whose profession is movement, few people are 'bodily aware'. Often, not until they become unwell, are hurt, or are perhaps surprised by a chance comment, 'you are so light on your feet', do they begin to observe themselves from a physically active point of view.

People do not always grow evenly, some may need a size 6 shoe on one foot and would be much happier if they could have a $5\frac{1}{2}$ size shoe on the other. A large number of people have one leg shorter than the other which often gives rise to low backache, the result of the uneconomical, unbalanced stance. To rectify this, the longer leg is bent at the knee as the body tries to overcome the imbalance by shortening the longer leg. People rarely notice this until it is pointed out to them. As riders they may also have not adjusted their leathers to accommodate for the discrepancy of leg length and so ride crooked.

It is nearly impossible to achieve a safe standard of riding, let alone a high standard in the absence of body awareness. How can a person who cannot feel a turn in or turn out at the hips respond to the command of an instructor 'open your hips'? There are many and varied schools teaching body awareness techniques, and of these the *Alexander* method is undoubtedly the best. The founder of the Alexander Technique was a medical doctor who appreciated, from an anatomical point of view, the things the human body could and, even more importantly, could not do. He also taught the necessity of influencing the central nervous system in order to teach students to realign their bodies. This ensured that each part rested correctly on the part immediately below, achieving perfect balance and changing permanently from previous uneconomical habit patterns to those that are both economical and efficient. The techniques must not be considered as the be all and end all of postural appreciation but they are a help to those who have no conception of body position in space. The techniques employed also achieve a heightened perception of the back, so important for the rider.

Preparation for the beginner at home

As a potential rider, or even an experienced rider, you should continue to improve 'body awareness'. The art of riding is to achieve an under-standing and awareness of the body language of your horse, a language transmitted to you via your eyes, hands, buttocks, inner thighs and lower legs. This language is based on sensations when each vibration, change of movement, attitude, and feel of the mass beneath you should impart a message. Then, through your heightened body awareness, you can translate and act upon these messages and learn to reply to the horse using your hands, buttocks, thighs, lower legs and voice.

In preparation, before even mounting a horse, you can practise learning to sense individual areas of your body as opposed to the whole. On a horse you are going to have to learn to appreciate the position of your horse's head through reins held in your fingers. Which direction does the sensation of pull come from? Are your hands being pulled up, exerting more pressure on the little fingers, or pulled down, exerting pressure on the index finger, or to one side, exerting pressure on the fingers of the right or left hand as the horse's head moves from side to side? Your fingers and thumbs must learn to tell you *exactly* what is happening with your horse's head, neck and forehand. When you become finger sensitive it is termed as having 'good hands'. However, you can only appreciate these minute message sensations if your grip on the reins is light – a rider with a rigid fist, gripping reins with whitened knuckles, is called a 'mutton fisted' rider.

To enable the finger sensations to register your shoulders must be relaxed, because tension between hand and neck will block the micro messages. Try sitting holding a pair of reins before you ever get on to a horse. Attach the reins to the leg of a table and then, closing your eyes, let your fingers talk to you. Tense your shoulders and relax them, exert pressure on the left rein, exert pressure on the right, and register the differing sensations. Train your buttocks by sitting on a hard chair – push all your weight through the left cheek, register, push all your weight through the right cheek, register. Learn to feel through your calf. Do this by standing on one leg and tapping the area of the calf which lies against the stirrup leather with the toe of your other foot. After all you are going to be tapping the sides of your horse, admittedly with your heel, but you can even learn that sensation by changing your own balanced position. Stand on a step facing outward with your knees slightly bent and lightly 'close' or push one heel against the riser. Do not look down while you are doing this – learn to move and feel without using your eyes. Should you have the misfortune to lose a stirrup while riding you have to find it again without using your eyes, particularly if you are speeding across country. There is no time to stop, look down, hold the leather with the appropriate hand and visually engage foot with iron. These simple activities enable you to begin to learn to record sensations from areas you have only previously recognised as being a part of your body if you have had the misfortune to hurt the area.

The foot

Your foot is a very important part of your vertical balance, even your squatting balance. Put a pair of irons on the floor and put your feet in them wearing your riding boots. Stand, with knees bent, and record the pressure that your body weight is exerting. Register the area of the sole of your foot where it is most comfortable for you to place the irons and from which you are getting the best 'balancing' messages. This will help when you first get on a horse and try to use your irons, for what they really become is a small floor. If you have a *safe* saddle horse in the tack room, sit on a saddle when it is off, rather than on the horse. This is how polo players learn 'stick and ball' by using a mechanical horse. There are a lot of mechanical horses about these days – jockeys use them to prepare their muscles for race riding and it is often possible to locate one and so experience the sensation of the riding position before you ever get onto a horse (Fig. 3.1).

To ride you need to improve the tone of your legs, particularly your ankle muscles. These are sited in the calf and down the outer side and front of the shin. Your body has to learn to function with hips and knees both slightly bent. All these movements are new learning skills because there is no other sport that demands skills comparable with sitting on a horse. It really is well worthwhile, however crude the preparation, to attempt to experience some of the new positions required before actually mounting an animal.

Repositioning the hip

The hip joints are sited at the junction of the lower body and thighs. To enable the rider to sit in the saddle these joints need to allow the thighs to turn out or externally rotate. This is normally described in equestrian

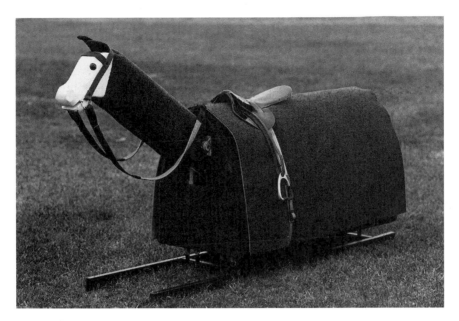

Fig. 3.1 A safe mechanical horse.

terms as 'opening the hips'. This outward turn at the hip joints, coupled with a slight lift of thigh towards the body (hip flexion), effectively cancels the natural extension lock mechanism of the knee, ingrained as essential, when the body is upright in standing, with weight passing through the feet. The suppression of this reflex 'knee lock' mechanism allows freedom of the lower leg, enabling it to perform the movements required, small, intricate, specialised excursions required to deliver, by contact with heel or spur, the commands or 'aids' to the sides of the ridden horse.

Long blunt spurs are KIND delivering signals with minimal knee excursion on the part of the rider, ensuring minimal disturbance to rider rhythm, and so saving on the equine energy which would be required if the horse needed to continually rebalance in response to position changes by the rider.

Further confusion occurs within normal natural balance mechanisms, because the rider's upper body must not angle forward in order to balance, as it would were the subject adopting a semi-squat position on the ground. The squat necessitates a similar hip repositioning to that of the mounted rider.

Maintenance of the riding position is much easier when a rider has learned the position of, and to balance on, the two bony projections or bumps sited within the buttocks, the *ischial tuberosities*. Add to these two other balance areas created by the muscles that lie between the inner thigh and the pelvis, often called the 'riders' muscles', taut when the rider is on the horse's back, due to thigh opening. It then becomes obvious, that for the rider, there is a natural, anatomically created base on which to sit, a diamond shaped base called *the seat*. To learn to use this base, allowing relaxed movements above and some activity below, is lesson number one.

If you are a new rider trying to learn the seat or a teacher trying to teach it, DO NOT HURRY. There is a saying *'do not run before you can walk'*, and for riders this should translate as *'only walk until you can sit'*.

The knee and ankle

Both the knee and ankle joints are *hinge joints*, that is they can only move in two planes. When a person stands the turning in or out of the leg and foot occurs at the hip joint. In the rider, because the knee is 'unlocked' secondary to hip position, the lower leg and ankle are able to turn (rotate) inward and outward at the knee enabling the closure of the heel to the horse's side.

Rider balance

The word *balance* denotes, in a physical sense, the equilibrium of body parts, in particular, the arrangement of the multi-jointed frame, the bony skeleton. Nature's arrangement is designed to minimise energy expenditure, particularly when associated with muscle activity. The bony skeleton according to John Gorman, an engineering specialising in mechanical sciences, is a miracle of design and the muscle arrangement ensures an effort-free, upright posture. Sitting poses a problem, for evolution has not adapted our frame to cope with long spells of sitting. This is a crucial difference between civilised man and the few tribes who are still, as were our ancestors, hunter-gatherers. One thing becomes obvious when we observe the range of movement available in the hip joints of these people. Natural man does not sit, he squats, allowing the bones of his back to retain their perfectly balanced design alignment, a situation only possible if full hip mobility is present. The lifestyle of natural man allows him to retain this necessary mobility.

The hip joint is described anatomically as a ball within a socket. The rounded ball-like head of the upper leg bone (the femur) moves within a half sphere, or saucer-shaped socket. This arrangement ensures a huge range of movement of the upper body on the legs, and a similar range of movement of the legs on the upper body. The design also allows the lower back to remain in a balanced state. Unfortunately, this freedom of movement at the hip joint can only be retained if the structures around the joint – ligaments, muscles and tendons – retain the elasticity with which they were endowed at birth and which remains during childhood. As we move around less, so the original elasticity diminishes and the movement range is reduced. In so-called civilised societies this reduction of movement has begun to occur by the age of 21 and the mobility of hip joints becomes increasingly reduced, unless addressed by appropriate exercises.

To enable a rider to balance, the hips *must be mobile.* A rider who, when positioned in the saddle, achieves a leather length and seat security enabling a hip angle of approximately 45°, achieves a near perfect lower back position which in turn assists upper body balance. The ability to balance is, of course, a combination of many factors, including the position of the neck and head, the use of the eyes, and specialist receptors sited in varying parts of the body, particularly in the soles of the feet. Balance in man is learned and occurs when, as children, we experiment in differing positions, eventually mastering those required for daily life. But learning need not end there, the ballet dancer achieves balance on point, the skater glides on narrow strips of laminated carbon. Riders can learn to balance using a child's space hopper (Figs 3.2 and 3.3).

To ride well man must find a position that suits his individual shape

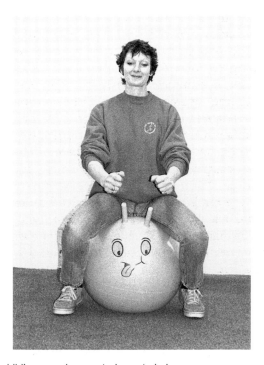

Fig. 3.2 Using a child's space hopper to learn to balance.

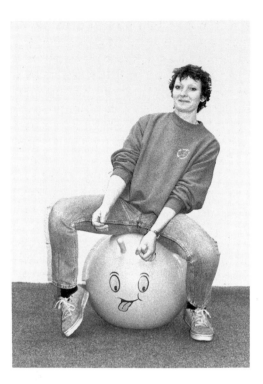

Fig. 3.3 Typical off-balance position adopted by novice riders.

and that also achieves a feeling of security. It is impossible for the new rider to achieve this, if, each time they ride, they encounter a new situation, for example, they are mounted on a different horse or use a different saddle. It is essential to learn balance on a similar horse using a similar saddle before attempting to change, as change necessitates adaptation to a set of different circumstances. Riding should be regarded as an art – the apprenticeship is long and painful and, as with the young horse, the learning takes time, a long time. The later in life a person starts to ride the longer it will take, but an aspiring rider need not be put off. In today's world too much is instant – patience, a considerable amount of patience, is required in order to ride well.

The aspiring rider must also understand, as previously stated, that man learns to balance and move the body utilising a series of interacting diagonals. For example, when walking, the left arm swings forward as the right leg moves forward, enhancing vertical balance. Vertical balance also necessitates contact between the soles of the feet and the ground and also a 'locked knee' during the weight-bearing phase of each step.

Despite much debate the human back *is* engineered for the upright posture. To achieve economical standing the feet need to be flat on the ground, so that they can impart the messages they are programmed to dispatch to all the other areas of the body. Loss of or disturbed foot function and reduced ground contact (often caused by thick soled shoes, high heels or arch supports) all disturb natural sensor mechanisms. These sensor mechanisms located within the foot are programmed not only to assist in the balance of the entire body, but also to warn all body parts of imminent impaction stresses. With this in mind, the previous suggestion is pertinent – that a rider should learn to balance on and to appreciate the input from the bars of a pair of stirrup irons before sitting on a horse.

Secondary to these new balance requirements the rider needs rhythm appreciation in order to harmonise with the movements of his or her mount. Movements created as the horse changes gait, circles, accelerates, decelerates, jumps, halts, and changes down from one pace to another. The smooth, apparently effortless accommodation on the part of a rider to all the changes created by the horse's movement takes time to achieve. Some people appear to have a natural ability for riding, while others struggle to improve and have endless lessons to no avail.

Children left to their own devices on a safe school master pony, riding without a saddle, harmonise rapidly and adopt a near perfect riding position in keeping with their shape and size. Although the child takes considerably longer to mature than the foal, the establishment of skills is similar, an often repeated action eventually becoming the accepted normal, the conscious thought previously required to perform the action no longer necessary. Most small children are fearless – this has problems when they associate with other species, so children should be taught a respect for the behaviour of, and the space required by, other species at an early age.

A great mistake made by some persons unfamiliar with horses is to imagine that a young child should be given a young pony, the idea being that the two will 'learn' and grow together. Put the situation in perspective – would you employ a three-year-old child to teach another three-year-old mathematics? Of course not, because neither of them fully understand the subject. There are exceptions to every rule but a learning child will benefit from an old, trusted pony who knows exactly what to do, enabling the child to learn to feel movements at all paces, to balance on the animal's back and to gradually respond to and move as one with the pony.

The most successful way to learn to ride as an adult is to ride bareback for short periods in the early learning stages, utilising a neck rein for security and balance, rather than using the reins and hanging on to the animal's mouth. Reconsider age – old ponies and horses rarely run away, young ones often do. Older, trusted school masters are not frightened if a child or adult falls off, young animals are frightened and may kick out, particularly if the rider falls under them.

Children can begin to sit on ponies before they can walk but they will not actually 'ride' until their legs are long enough to firstly achieve security, giving them balance independent of their hands, and secondly to allow them to administer leg 'aids'. Children that learn to ride bareback will eventually be able to adapt to any saddle, because their balance on an independently moving being has become so automatically tuned (it has become reflex) that they go with, rather than against, any movement that may be encountered. Technical refinements can come later. The same applies to an adult – to sit on a horse bareback with a neck rein in safe surroundings will enhance the ability to learn balance quicker than by any other method. All the refinements can, as with the child, be attempted later. To envisage this, think how badly you drove a car during your first lesson. Improvement was gradual then you were eventually able to coordinate, without any conscious thought, a chain of reactions never previously attempted. As you began to coordinate you achieved the movements necessary without them being jerky and without exerting excessive strength, so a series of smooth, independent actions became an automatic normal. You had established your driving reflexes. It is exactly the same when learning to ride. Watch a pupil experiencing trot for the first time – everything moves. Then look at an accomplished rider, the movements of the accomplished rider have become subtle and the rhythm of movement effortless.

The young child has no preconceived ideas and may remain unpoised for slightly longer than the learning adult, because maturation and learning tend to occur in fits and starts. Do not be disappointed in an apparent lack of progression in either a young horse, a young child or when a rider *or* horse is attempting a new discipline.

Seat and hands

The terms 'seat' and 'hands' deserve explanation. Professional dancers learn body awareness by following an established, proven method. Nearly every dancer first learns basic classical ballet, they then progress and diversify. The Classical methods of riding, developed mainly in Europe for the education of both horse and rider, have never been surpassed. Once the basics of these teachings have been mastered there are of course many variations. These may necessitate changes, perhaps of leather length, saddle shape, saddle type or rider position, necessary to help horse and rider comply with the demands of diverse equestrian activities.

To ride a horse and achieve a good, stable seat requires total reposi-tioning of the lower limbs. Hip, knee and ankle joints must align in a manner which, in standing, would be considered by the brain to be both uneconomic and dangerous. The muscle groups and joints have to learn a new, coordinated pattern.

To maintain the 'seat' the muscles involved, just like the lower limb muscles, have to learn new interactions. The body balance mechanisms, normally needing intimate connections from the ground, through the soles of the entire foot, have to learn to accept signals from only the area of the foot in contact with the saddle bar and to interconnect with the signals generated as a result of sitting on the new *base*.

Stirrups should not be regarded as a means for staying on, rather they are an accessory to assist in the maintenance of lower leg position. In the Classical School all the aids above ground are performed without stirrups, and Mark Todd rode the second half of a cross country at Badminton without his stirrups after a leather broke. The stirrup itself is a comparatively late invention in equestrianism, saddle pads having been described in approximately 500 BC and before, but accounts of stirrups or 'irons' do not appear until 577 AD and even later in Britain. When William the Conqueror invaded in 1066 AD he is supposed to have won the Battle of Hastings due to the fact his army had stirrups and the British did not.

For comfort and communication the rider's hands should work as a matched pair. This is difficult for people who are neither naturally ambidextrous nor have hand sensitivity. To many people hands are useful tools on the end of the arms but hands need to be trained to feel and to interpret subtle signals delivered to the fingers, palms and thumbs. Only by activating dormant pathways can a rider learn to communicate, via the reins and bit, with the mouth, head, neck and forelimbs of the horse. Luck, in the design of the equine mouth, allows us to place a bit in the gap between two sets of teeth, the *incisors* and the *premolars* so that we can communicate, via the reins and bit, between the rider's hands and the horse's mouth.

Much descriptive terminology is used to try to establish a meaningful appreciation of the term 'good hands'. Think of holding a silk cord. Think of egg shells. Zenephon stated 'it is as well to get into the habit of sitting quiet and utterly avoid touching him (the horse) with any other parts than those which we use in securing a firm seat.' Nuno Olivera, perhaps to be regarded as the modern day Zenephon, stated 'the rider who is not properly in the saddle, supple and as one with the horse, can never achieve independence.' He goes on to say 'it is only with a good position and supple horse that the rider may succeed in stabilising his hands for communication and thus being certain of never pulling on his horse's mouth.' He continues 'a good piece of advice to all who want to ride well and who wish to acquire a good position would be to do *gymnastic exercises*, those which will give suppleness, ease and sureness in riding.'

Good hands are available to all once the rider's seat is secure and independent of their hands. This is only possible if the rider is supple, trained by appropriate gymnastic exercises. From the remarks of these two great masters it must be obvious that you do not hold on by the reins and an aspiring rider should teach themselves tactile appreciation when both off and on the horse. Communication through light touch is essential. Sadly many horses, particularly those whose preparation has been rushed, have not been schooled (taught) in a manner which enables this subtle interaction to occur. Always remember, *it is as hard for the horse to learn as it is for the rider*. Time is essential, and the learning and retention of lessons do not occur in days, weeks or months, it takes years. Ballet dancers start at five years old and begin to dance when they reach the age of eighteen or twenty one. Schools devoted to producing sportsmen will not admit children after the age of seven or eight and aim for their eventual participation as an athlete ten years later. Short cuts lead to poor performance and to disappointment. Besides tactile and balance conceptual learning, your off horse preparation should also involve some form of active exercise. If your horse is busy working in his gym, the arena, preparing to learn to carry you, the rider, the least that you can do is to engage in some sort of general body preparation.

Muscle recoordination

Muscles around the human hip joint are programmed to coordinate in every day life for the activities involved in walking, running, sitting, and rising from sitting. All hip activities involve the gluteal or buttock muscles known as *hip extensors*. The muscle ileopsoas, lying inside the pelvis in front of the lower back, passes forward to join an internal groin muscle, known as a *hip flexor*. These two sets of muscles work together as equal and opposites. They are assisted in hip control by a group positioned between the inner thigh and the front bar of the pelvis – these are adductor muscles and are known to riders as the *rider's muscle*. This group, previously described as being a part of the rider's *seat base*, interact with two partners within the buttock that work as abductors.

When man sits on a horse, bare back, or on a saddle, all these groups have to reorganise their interactions, learning to allow the upper body to remain upright for the most part but balanced on hips that are opened, and with the lower leg no longer required to lock at the knee.

The back

Anatomically, the back stretches from the base of the skull to the pelvis, divided into three distinct areas – the neck, the mid back, the lower back. The whole is balanced upon the pelvis, which in turn balances on the hips.

The lower back is the epicentre of balance and should, contrary to general belief, be *stable* NOT *mobile*. All movement starts from a fixed point. A stable, strong, lower lumbar area allows the upper body the freedom to adjust without tension or fatigue. A rider who has an unstable lower back will waste endless energy trying to maintain balance by utilising muscles rather than learning poise.

The shoulders

The arms hang from a bone arrangement similar in design to a milkmaid's yoke. The relaxation of the arms and their movement on the body from shoulder joint to fingers is governed by the degree of tension or relaxation within the muscles of the yoke. As those muscles spread upward, supporting the neck and head, these structures are also interdependent upon the levels of tension or relaxation in the shoulder complex.

The head

Amongst their many duties, the structures of the head, in particular the lower jaw, are intimately concerned with balance. A rigid, set jaw creates a stiff neck, leading to tension and immobility throughout the entire body. In the young child, whose movement coordination is not yet 'hard wired', relaxation is comparatively easy; for more mature riders and those lacking body awareness, the learning curve to achieve the necessary relaxation for riding takes longer.

Development for ridden skills in the horse

Play

Babies of all species learn through play. Despite being born equipped with senses and assets needed for survival the foal is no different; it merely has fewer skills to learn than babies of some other species, notably predators. Fortunately, despite being the most perceptive of all the domesticated species, careful exposure to new experiences will, in most horses, diffuse their natural instinctive reactions and replace these with the behavioural responses required by man. However, the thinking rider, owner or groom must *never* become complacent, for although controlled, the fear reaction, described as an instinctive reaction, can never be totally eliminated. Domesticated animals have had to acquire behavioural patterns different which in the wild would be inappropriate. Despite interaction with man for the past 6000 years, during which time the horses of today have emerged, no documented genetic imprint responses are apparent. Every horse we handle, every horse we break in, can revert to in-built, natural responses – those of a prey species. These are:

- flee if you are frightened;
- fight if you cannot;
- attack with teeth and/or heels if pain joins fear.

Imprinting

The earlier the foal learns that man is *not* an enemy, the better. A new programme aimed at the establishment of early intercommunication has become termed 'imprinting'. A contented mare, in surroundings she considers safe will convey her feelings to her foal. It is then within a few hours of birth that communication between man and foal should begin. If the job is well done the foal will learn to subdue its natural fear of this strange, two-legged being, towering above it and with an offensive smell. If handled with confidence and extreme care, things which in the natural state would cause fear will become the accepted normal. Indeed, if with gentle finger massage, man mimics the licking sensation of the mare given when the foal is first born the foal will not only accept humans but will also associate them with pleasure.

It is a good idea to expose a young foal to the following:

- The early fitting of a head collar (always use an adjustable nose strap as foals grow fast and I have seen animals unable to graze or suck because the nose piece of the head collar has become so tight the foal cannot open its mouth).
- A light roller to mimic a girth.
- Legs felt and, as balance becomes stable, feet picked up.

Provided all these activities are performed within a secure, stable environment all will gradually be accepted and resistance to shoeing or to saddle and bridle in later life, will be almost non-existent.

In the early days immediately following foaling these activities should be carried out daily in a similar manner and, if possible, by the same smelling person, until total confidence is apparent in the young animal. The foal then comes forward to greet the person, rather than trying to back away to hide behind or cower by its dam. Gradually other people can be introduced and the foal's experiences should be widened to include other animals. (I have owned horses who had obviously never seen a cow and I have had an interesting ride as a result!) Most thoroughbred foals travel early in life to return from the studs where they were born, but it is a good idea to put a foal born at home in a horsebox or trailer with its dam early on. This is not necessarily to travel but once again in order that it experiences a new, totally alien situation that it will meet in later life.

As the foal grows and is led, perhaps to and from pasture with its dam, or if it appears in the show ring, take care that it does not out walk the handler. The restraint applied, even if it is being led from a centrally placed D ring, will tend to make the animal turn its head slightly towards the handler, feeling as it does so increased pressure both behind the ears and on the nose. The head turn is usually to the left as most animals are led from their near or left side. This left head turn becomes imprinted in the foal's brain, recorded as 'pressure behind the ears, pressure on the nose, turn the head slightly left'. This posture will be adopted whenever pressure in those areas is felt. *The handler has programmed in a brain response or 'imprint'.* As the animal develops and begins to wear tack in preparation to be ridden at two or three years the bridle is put on and the animal feels pressure behind the ears and on the nose. Immediately there is a marginal turn of head and neck to the left. *Thought must accompany every new lesson.* For example, when the animal is released in a field it should be taught to walk through the gate and stand quietly while the head collar is removed, rather than be allowed to barge through the gate and fight to get loose.

Early living

Whenever possible, foals should be given a large, preferably undulating, space in which to run, where they can gallop to run out of energy, slowing down under control rather than skidding to a stop when reaching the boundary fence. An undulating field is beneficial as it teaches balance: 'as sure footed as a mountain pony' is an old maxim. Mountain ponies scramble up and down the sides of hills and gallops on steep slopes, learning a mass of invaluable balance reactions and building muscles not utilised on the flat. The best polo ponies have cut cattle running behind their working mothers. Never forget, to confine a young animal is to be unkind, not kind. All young animals learn through play so to deny them these experiences will lengthen their eventual training programme. A horse that has not learned to balance unridden will find it very hard to balance when encumbered with both rider weight and when meeting uneven ground for the first time.

Because horses are herd animals by nature, unless one of the herd turns out to be a bully, the animals are much happier if turned out in the company of other horses. In addition, as the young learn from the old, even a retired gelding or an old mare is better than nothing for company. Many of these herd associated skills are disregarded by man, but today we hear of elephant families dying out because slaughter of the old animals for ivory has left the younger members without the necessary knowledge to survive. Teenage elephants try to look after younger members but do not know the migration trails, water holes or safe areas in storm conditions. Horses are no different, even though they have been domesticated by man, and difficult horses (those hard to handle, frightened of traffic, or slow to learn when working in long reins) respond if you put an experienced horse alongside the problem animal. Some difficulties are rapidly overcome, particularly those associated with traffic, noise, loading and being caught.

Worming

A regular worm programme is as essential for foals as it is for older horses. Worm damage causes irreversible changes in the mesentery of the intestines, reducing the area available for nutrient absorption. This situation may stop an animal achieving its full potential because activity demands increased uptake of all foods. If this uptake is poor the animal will not be able to service its musculo-skeletal requirements.

Feet

On soft grass paddocks feet do not wear or harden. Remember that wild horses live on vast, arid plains. Animals turned out on mountains rarely require their feet to be trimmed because the terrain naturally trims. Recent studies of horses in the wild have shown that they square off their toes. This observation has led, particularly in America, to a new shoeing method (four point shoeing) shaping the foot in a manner which allows the horse to break over a squared-off toe. Regular attention to your horse's feet is necessary throughout life. The quality of the wall of the hoof, the sole and the state of the frog are all indicators of general health. Dry brittle hooves, contracted heels or dry and cracking soles indicate a dietary deficiency. Careful consideration is necessary before rushing out buying yet another additive when a horse develops poor quality feet. Consult your vet or use a help line, such as that provided by Natural Animal Feeds.

Training

As the young animal grows decisions need to be made regarding training. Many of these depend upon breed. For example, the racing thoroughbred has been selectively bred to do that which comes naturally, to run very fast for a very short distance early in life. This is exactly what the animal would do in the wild, the only difference being a light weight upon its back. Training needs to address the weight bearing and to ensure that both frame and muscles are prepared adequately for the short race, but not over stressed by too much hard galloping. Other breeds mature more slowly. The large warmbloods look strong but do not reach skeletal maturity until they are 7 or even 8 years old. Many are ruined by being asked to perform at an exacting level when far too young. Reference to texts of approximately 30 years ago show that few animals other than flat bred thoroughbreds were broken in or ridden before the age of four and a half and not expected to compete until their sixth year. Sadly few horses are given the necessary amount of time to develop. This has led to a considerable rise in skeletal and soft tissue injuries and a loss of performance at a very early age in many.

Chapter 4
Diet

Horses trained from their field are probably amongst the most successful, this fact borne out by the impressive results of the New Zealand and Australian three day event horses in recent years. All are trained from the field.

Recent observations demonstrate that, given the choice, the natural horse grazes on poor quality grasses (providing bulk fibre) and derives its vitamins and minerals from grazed herbal sources and by licking mineral-rich rocks. Most wild animals follow migratory routes which pass mineral-rich rock outcrops. There they may spend 2–3 days licking the rocks in order to supply their bodies with sufficient minerals to last them for many months.

Horses turned out to pasture may dig the soil and eat dirt. They are seeking the nutrients they instinctively realise their systems are lacking. When the horse was an agricultural necessity it was common practice to cut a sod of turf and put it into the animal's water bucket because the minerals in the soil dissolved into the water. Water soluble nutrients are easily absorbed. It was also normal practice to feed root vegetables such as swedes, mangle worzles (a vegetable of the past) or carrots, all of which store minerals and vitamins in their tuberous roots.

Under natural conditions the horse grazes for up to 15 hours a day, allowing a continual and slow process of digestion and absorption to occur. The animal may also walk up to 20 miles a day, and the gut motion created aids digestion and the passage of food. What do you do with a horse that is showing signs of colic? You walk the animal, not just to prevent it rolling but to encourage the normal movement of the intestines (called peristalsis) to re-establish in the areas of the gut where the activity has changed, become irregular, and where blockage may occur.

Despite the pronouncements of many feed experts we are still a long way from understanding nutrition in any species. Look at the human literature, fats in, fats out, this mineral, that mineral, more of this, less of that. The information continuously changes with the most recent usually in total contradiction to the information supplied by a previous bulletin. The horse evolved in areas most suited to its needs, but despite searching world-wide I can find no analysis of the minerals present in those soils, of the plants available, or of the composition of the water.

Why should the horse need probiotics? Do any of us really need to change a gut flora that has evolved, apparently successfully, over millions of years? One thing is quite certain – most horses are grossly over supplemented. Scientific studies indicate that some of the best equine athletes are fed a very simple diet, one consisting of good hay, free range grazing and good quality oats or corn. A recent example confirms this: an endurance horse was continuously unwell for two seasons and, despite being given every additive, balanced feeds and supplementation, the animal tied up, was muscle sore, appeared tired, thin, and under-nourished, had scant bad smelling urine and failed every vet check at competition. It was suggested that the animal be trained from the field, and its diet radically changed by being simplified. In addition to free grazing, carrots and good quality chaff were offered three times a day and the supplementation of a mineral mix incorporated. Rock salt was left at the water trough and a level tablespoon of copper sulphate was added to the field trough if there were any signs of green algae. This worked out as a level spoonful a month if it was sunny, less as it became colder, in a large field tank. This is an old remedy for keeping field troughs algae-free, described in early farming books c. 1800, and allows the horse access to minute amounts of copper, an element essential for efficient respiratory function. During the next season the horse in question ran 725 miles in long distance competition and was trained 100 miles a week. The animal gained his 1000 mile award, was runner up in three major trophy races and third in two others. The owner has stated that she was frightened to tell the vets what the animal was being fed as so many of the other horses she was beating were on high performance rations and she felt it would go against her if she confessed to such a simple diet. In three months the horse was a changed animal, bright, alert, well-muscled, and results showed it was competing to a high performance level. In six months the animal was unrecognisable and the rider was being asked where she had found such a marvellous new horse.

Understanding rations and supplements

A balanced, naturally achieved diet *should* contain all essential nutrients, electrolytes, minerals and vitamins. Natural horse and natural man both survived without supplementation. There is a belief that supplementation will enhance performance although there is little scientific evidence to support the theory unless there are known dietary deficiencies, in which case supplementation may be advisable.

Unfortunately, modern farming methods, geared to intensive production, have changed the structure of the soil. Many areas, originally worked on a rotation system, with replenishment of macro and micro minerals achieved by the use of animal waste as fertiliser, are now shown to be deficient of many of their original components and it follows that plants or herbage grown under such conditions will themselves contain less nutrients. These factors have led to the attempted development of 'balanced food' accompanied by an explosion in additive use.

If supplementation is introduced great care must be taken not to mix products and also to ensure the instructions regarding dosage are followed. The requirements of a healthy body are finely balanced. Too much is as dangerous as too little because an excess of any dietary component cannot be stored against need. The body will only extract what is actually required to service immediate demand and the excess will either be excreted, wasting energy in the process, or sent to the liver (particularly if the body is unable to recognise the substance), leading, in some circumstances, to toxicity. The exact daily requirement of minerals and vitamins is still unknown and suggested levels are a calculated guestimate.

The body manufactures many of its required components, either from the ingredients contained in the nutritional intake or, in the case of vitamin D, from sunlight, provided there is adequate exposure of the skin to sunlight throughout the year. Extra vitamin D (by injection or some other method) is totally contra-indicated unless advised by a veterinarian. *Excess is toxic,* causing calcification problems in blood vessels, tendons and ligaments.

Selenium and vitamin E are constantly discussed, however an adequate sufficiency of both should be present in all good quality hay. *Excess selenium is toxic,* causing severe problems in the hoof and sometimes in the skin. While certain areas of the world are selenium-deficient horses are not naturally attracted to these areas. For domesticated animals, because soil analysis pinpoints such deficiencies, it is unlikely that a horse would be offered a selenium-deficient diet. No farmer can grow crops successfully on totally selenium-deficient land so farmers supplement, in order to ensure sufficient selenium is present in the soil, thereby ensuring that the plants growing in the area extract the amount they require.

The following list is of the major vitamins and minerals. All have specific functions common to both man and the horse.

Vitamins

Vitamin A

- Required for absorption
- Stored in the liver

- Required for enhancing vision in dim light
- Maintains the health of certain cells, in particular those lining the airways (the mucosal epithelium)
- *Excess is toxic*

Vitamin B₁

- Involved in carbohydrate metabolism

Vitamin B₂

- Involved in energy metabolism

Vitamin B₆

- Involved in protein metabolism

Vitamin B₁₂

- Involved in the formation of red blood cells
- Involved in energy production, particularly the synthesis of DNA and RNA

Vitamin C

- Involved in the absorption of iron

Vitamin D

- Regulates calcium and phosphate metabolism
- Assists in the mineralisation of bone

Vitamin E

- Reacts with selenium
- Regulates calcium and phosphorus absorption

Vitamin K

- Assists in the formation of essential blood clotting agents
- *Large amounts are toxic*

Minerals

Calcium

- Required for the development of bones and teeth
- Required for muscle contraction
- Required for the transmission of nerve impulses (messages)
- Involved in the maintenance of the rhythm of the heart
- Involved in cell membrane permeability

Chlorine

- Involved in the digestive processes in the stomach
- Assists in the acid–base balance
- Is the main anion in extracellular fluid

Chromium

- Assists in the formation of chemical energy
- Assists in protein synthesis

Copper

- Involved in the synthesis and absorption of iron to produce haemo-globin
- Involved in electron transport
- Involved in the construction of nerve insulation (the sheath)

Fluorine

- Required to prevent decay in bones and teeth

Iron

- Required for the formation of haemoglobin and myoglobin
- A constituent of oxidative enzymes

Magnesium

- Required for muscle and nerve response (irritability)
- Required for carbohydrate metabolism
- A constituent of teeth and bone

Manganese

- Involved in the formation of bone
- Involved in enzyme activity for many processes

Phosphorus

- Required for bone and tooth formation
- Required for cell permeability
- Required for the metabolism of carbohydrates and fats
- Involved in the storage and release of ATP

Potassium

- Required for nerve and muscle response
- Is the principal cation of the intracellular fluid
- Involved in both water and acid–base balance
- Involved in the maintenance of heart rhythm
- Involved in protein synthesis

Selenium

- An antioxidant
- *Excess is toxic*

Sodium

- Involved in the regulation of nerve function
- Involved in the regulation of muscle contraction
- Involved in both water and the acid–base balance
- The principal cation in extracellular fluid

Sulphur

- A vital constituent of proteins and especially important in cartilage
- Involved in detoxification
- Involved in many complex cellular interactions

Zinc

- A vital constituent of enzymes
- Necessary for the completion of many complex body interactions.

   The list of vitamins and minerals is not a full list for, as science progresses and analysis of cells and their components continues, 'new' elements appear in the complex formulae describing cell metabolism. Supplementation is therefore a very complex subject. Food produced from natural sources contains a better balance of nutrients than that produced by intensive chemical cultivation. This is demonstrated by the current trend towards organic production.

Electrolytes

A horse that is provided with adequate fresh water and a block of natural salt (as opposed to a man-made lick) will obtain adequate electrolytes from its diet. Only if excessive sweating occurs, due to climatic conditions or exercise stress, should electrolyte supplementation be necessary.

A horse cannot store electrolytes against need. Electrolytes maintain the fluid balance within the tissues and need to be present in exact amounts. Supplementation, particularly if the electrolytes are provided 'dry' upsets this *steady state* between intra- and extracellular fluids. In the case of dry supplementation, in order to suspend the often unnecessary electrolytes fluid will be drawn from intracellular areas, creating unnecessary energy loss secondary to the fluid imbalance created.

Protein

Protein is the basic building block required for cell and therefore tissue construction. As exercise demands increase, protein intake will require adjustment. You may choose to address the need by introducing hay containing a higher protein level or by increasing the levels of protein in hard feed. In all cases any increase should be gradual. It is worth remembering that any change of hay, horsehage or similar bulking foods requires careful consideration because each will vary widely in its nutritional value. These variations are due to the food source, time of year when made, moisture content when the grasses were cut. Far too many horses 'tie up' following the arrival of a new batch of bulking feed. In the days when sufficient hay could be stored to last the winter, and enough of that batch was still in the barn to be fed the following autumn, a similar nutritional level could be maintained throughout the year and neither way the hay too rich. Constant changes create digestive problems, these leading in turn to loss of condition and reduced performance levels.

While considering protein intake it follows that if exercise demands decrease, so protein levels should be reduced. Over-feeding, using high quality feeds, is often more disastrous than slightly under-feeding. The most important factor for the horse is always adequate, good quality feed, free of both dust and moulds. Moulds are not confined to hay alone; oats get musty in damp conditions as do all bagged balanced ration feeds.

Carbohydrates

Energy required for muscle activity is released when carbohydrate from the fibre in a horse's food is metabolised. Feeding bulk food is important due to the design of the equine digestive system and the in-built requirement of the horse to chew. Well bulked food, that is concentrates mixed with chop (chaff), will encourage the horse to chew slowly, grinding the food matter and ensuring an efficient start to digestion and the subsequent metabolic absorption processes. It has been calculated that a kilo of bulked food will require the horse to chew approximately 5300 times, whereas a kilo of concentrates will only be chewed around 1000 times. The latter creates a bolus or block of food, which passes rapidly first into the stomach and then into the intestines, rather than the preferable continual steady flow of food, achieved by the slow passage of bulked food.

In common with human athletes the type of competition and individual metabolism will, to a degree, dictate nutritional requirements. Horses are creatures of habit and perform best if given their rations at a similar time each day. Designed to eat from the ground they are able to digest better if floor fed. This method also reduces considerably the risk of the inhalation of dust, which can happen particularly if dry hay is pulled from a rack or net.

Weight

Weighing horses has become a popular method for calculating food requirements. Obviously the more energy burnt the more replacement required. All racing stables talk about their horses racing weights and most are weighed after a race to record weight lost, the amount lost being an indicator, not only of the animal's fitness but also of the effort it put into that particular race.

Unfortunately only time will tell you, the owner, rider or trainer, the animal's ideal weight. These weights can only be calculated on performance records during training and competition. Weighing a horse will also give you some indication if an overweight horse is beginning to change flab to muscle, but nothing beats an expert's eye.

The fat horse

If the horse is overweight you need to try to reduce the excess weight while maintaining appetite satisfaction. The best way to achieve this is to increase workload gradually, and, as appetite increases, to feed good, low-energy roughage (hay). This given 'ad lib' will fulfil the hunger the animal is experiencing. Due to the low nutritional quality of the hay and the body's demand for fuel, the body will be forced to utilise any excess fat stores and to convert these into the energy required for work.

A thin horse

A horse who comes up in poor condition, that is light or thin, and in need of increased flesh is obviously different from the fat horse. A horse with no reserves of energy finds even light work a big drain. With these type of horses, the conditioning programme has to proceed very slowly. Check for worms, check the teeth, have a blood test and do not just hope things will improve. Amongst other reasons for a veterinary examination is the fact that you can find out if your horse, like so many today, has developed a stomach ulcer. It has been discovered that stressed horses, just like stressed humans develop gastric (stomach) ulcers. No amount of additives, magic potions or probiotics will cure an ulcer. Specialist drugs are required. They are very successful and many previously miserable horses thrive following a course of treatment.

A horse in training who is gaining weight

If an animal in serious training continues to gain weight it is obviously being fed rations containing more nutrients than are required for the current work load. There are two choices: either decrease the energy content of the ration or increase the work load. Once again, in order to satisfy appetite it may be necessary to add some good hay, but of low nutritional value. If the animal is eating its bedding, should it be on straw, change to paper or shavings, or spray the straw with a disinfectant to make it unpalatable.

The horse in training who is losing weight

The horse in training that is losing considerable weight is either burning more energy than that supplied in the rations or it is unwell. These cases are more difficult to deal with because the animal may already be being given enough food to satisfy its appetite. In this case cut back the intensity and requirements of the exercise and build more slowly toward the final goal. Sometimes introducing an extra feed last thing at night makes a big difference. Four or five small feeds rather than two or three large feeds will often tempt poor eaters.

The horse in work who is maintaining its weight

When a horse maintains its optimum weight and works satisfactorily this shows that the rations are correctly balanced for the horse's work requirements. However, this sometimes poses a problem because people are always looking for improved performance and there is a tendency to try to increase the ration in order to achieve this. Any random change should be avoided: the horse is maintaining its weight so is obviously receiving adequate energy from its food. Improved performance requires not just extra rations but also increased activity and training.

Feed change

If you do decide to make changes in the horse's feed it is essential to do it slowly because the digestive system becomes accustomed to particular foods. To change rapidly to another diet is a remedy for disaster. The annual change from old to new hay is a prime example. New hay, that is hay less than six months old, should be introduced by mixing some with the old hay and increasing the amount of new hay gradually over a two to three week period. In one year the spring and summer in Britain were very wet and the quality of traditional hay and haylidge differed widely from that made the year before. Because of these differences problems occurred with horses 'tying up' when they were introduced rapidly to the new hay.

It is sensible to feed a horse at the same time each day and studies have suggested that food arriving at regular intervals can improve a horse's performance by up to 40%.

Other dietary factors

Only time, performance evaluation, and the reading of an animal's condition will tell what food best suits each particular animal; some cannot tolerate certain types of grain while others become unwell if sugar beet is added to their rations. Unfortunately one of the major problems of today's balanced feeds is that, while they must contain the protein, mineral, fibre levels printed on the label, there is no guarantee that the ingredients come from the same source for each new batch.

Feeding a horse is part of *the art of husbandry*, and horses do not get fit without both food and activity. A rider once asked me, in response to a question regarding the work load of her horse, 'Why does he need to work in order for me to compete? The information on the food package states that the food will keep him fit and healthy.'

Having addressed diet, three other factors should be considered before serious training starts: worming, injections and blood testing. While riders rarely require worming, unless they have visited areas of the world in which the human worms are common, far too many grooms and riders neglect their own injections. It is *essential* to ensure that tetanus protection is regularly updated. Human blood tests should not be neglected as an anaemic rider is no use to a fit horse.

Worming

Before starting on a training programme it is sensible to worm your animal. Indications are that many horses are becoming resistant to the conventional programmes, but the offices of all veterinary practitioners will give up to date information on the subject.

Injections

A horse should be up to date with all the necessary injections before starting work. Many horses feel very 'off colour' for several days after their flu jabs, some develop mild coughs, even a runny nose. They must be given time to recover fully, two to three days at least, before going back to or starting work.

Blood

In any training programme the regular monitoring of the profile of cell populations via a blood test is essential. The blood can be likened to a barometer, giving pointers to the current state of health. Of the many pointers available from a blood analysis is the level of haemoglobin.

Haemoglobin is a special oxygen transport chemical, comprising 33% of every single red blood cell. The haemoglobin is able to attract oxygen molecules from the lungs and, following their delivery to the body tissues, collect carbon dioxide for eventual excretion.

Cell conception is very hard and, when you learn that the average thousand pound horse has approximately 510 trillion blood cells circulating in its blood system at any one time, you may be forgiven for beginning to wonder how on earth you can ever train this animal to perfection. Unlike some other cell types, red blood cells do not reproduce themselves but are actually produced from a complex series of interactions in the marrow of the long bones and also in the liver and spleen.

The spleen is very important to the exercising horse and can perhaps be compared to a rather large sponge full of blood cells. It serves as a container for healthy red blood cells and a recycling yard for those that have finished their life cycle. Just as the kidneys are able to recycle certain components and return them for reuse so specialist capillaries in the spleen itself are able to break down used and dying blood cells. In an impressive display of efficiency iron is taken from the decaying cells and transported back to the bone marrow and to the liver for reuse, being incorporated into new cells as they are manufactured.

Under strenuous exercise conditions a horse is often described as having got its 'second wind'. The second wind occurs due to a contraction of the spleen which releases a huge number of red cells into the circulating blood. Their presence achieves an immediate improved oxygen delivery, provided the lungs are functioning properly. The contraction of the spleen is a reflex response to the body's demands.

The efficiency of the red cells for oxygen delivery and carbon dioxide removal and the number present in the blood are critical to equine performance. It is during interval training that vital signals are generated to enhance the production of red cells. As the horse becomes fatigued a state of oxygen debt occurs and demand for oxygen rises. Specialist systems recognise the necessity for more oxygen. The only way to ensure the arrival of extra oxygen to the oxygen depleted tissues is to increase the number of blood cells available, both to carry the oxygen required for muscle activity and to remove the carbon dioxide created. Only by increasing the work demand can this occur. It cannot be achieved by pumping in varied tonics and other substances said to 'improve' the production of red cells. It is certainly true that extra components may be necessary in cases of dietary deficiency or metabolic upset, in which case these components are normally given by injection, and may include extra protein, iron, copper and cobalt, all of which are among the raw materials required for the manufacture of red blood cells.

A normal, well-balanced diet should contain all the necessary components in adequate amounts: this is what the term 'balanced diet' means. The mix, however it is supplied (as nuts, cubes or mixes), is supposed to contain everything required to build the cells of all the tissues and to supply 'fuel' for those tissues to use.

As the condition of your horse improves you will notice a change in its haemoglobin levels because the bone marrow, liver and spleen have stepped up production in response to demand. A horse that is getting less exercise demands less oxygen, and lack of demand reduces the number of red cells in production.

The body is very economical and does not waste energy in the production of anything non-essential. Formation of all components is controlled by the demands of training. This applies to all the body systems and therefore a continued level of exercise, once fitness for the required task has been achieved, maintains a steady state, enabling the animal to continue to compete at a reasonable level.

The blood test can also demonstrate if there has been a massive muscle breakdown in response either to exercise or trauma, if an infection is present, or if the animal is recovering from infection. There is a host of vital information available from a blood test. Another reason for monitoring blood profiles is that a tissue under stress, before it breaks down, releases certain chemicals which can be analysed as another diagnostic aid. The reading of the blood test and reporting on the health picture it gives is the job of a highly qualified veterinarian. Money used to pay for blood tests is never wasted; tests should be taken at regular intervals and these intervals should be discussed with your veterinarian during any training programme.

Chapter 5
The Memory of Cells

As knowledge of cellular behaviour advances many of the training protocols used by our forebears are being rationalised. Scientists have isolated some of the requirements at cellular level, of the varied tissues. These requirements, if met by appropriate nutrition and level of activity, enables cells to function properly and to stand, without breakdown, the demands created by these activities. First, the tissues adapt to low level exertion, then remodel in order to counteract extra stresses encountered during intensive training. However, there is still a great deal to be understood in the science of cellular behaviour.

One important point that has become clear is the fact that cells and therefore tissues which are constructed from the cells, have a memory and a huge variety of information can be stored against requirement following exposure to and experience of complex stress patterns created during activity. In Chapter 3, the necessity to learn to feel, to balance, to communicate through touch, were discussed, these 'gross' learning curves requiring repetition to establish reflex responses. Cellular memory can be envisioned in the same way.

It may help to grasp the idea of cellular memory by visualising a football team, each player has his own specific task, each player needs, by doing his particular job, to complement the performance of the whole to the very best of his ability. To achieve this each player, dependent upon his position on the field must learn, by constantly practising, the moves he will require. He is training in order to combat every situation likely to arise in his particular sector when playing as a team member.

Envisage the different body tissues as the individual players, while the team represents the body. Just like each footballer, every tissue needs to be trained to play its part to complement the whole. Each tissue will have specific requirements, and each needs to be exposed to a wide variety of eventual demands, enabling it to store, in its 'memory', the characteristics of each experience. None of this 'team work' would occur without the interlinkage of the body systems described in Chapter 2.

Bone adaptation to training

In order to avoid breakdown the bone frame (skeleton) must be able to withstand

- Traction exerted by working muscles
- Ground impaction forces
- Functional load bearing (this last incurring increased demand in the case of overweight subjects)

It has been clearly established that bone is capable of an adaptive response to loading. What is unclear is which methods of training are the most effective to achieve the required response. Improved methods for diagnosis demonstrate considerably more bone related athletic injuries than previously recognised in both man and horse.

Training bone

Despite the fact that structural failure of bone in either man or the horse is catastrophic remarkably little research has been directed to determine the appropriate methods for conditioning bone. Mechanical loading of bone *in vitro* for both species has demonstrated the levels of cyclical loading required to shatter bone and, useful though this research may be to some, and while the experimental bone was once part of a living being, in the laboratory it no longer has the ligaments, tendons, muscles or a blood supply enjoyed *in vivo*. Such experiments are purely of academic interest rather than having an immediate practical outcome.

Factors affecting bone remodelling

Activity creates a degree of functional skeletal loading, the bones of the skeleton adapting to avoid structural failure. Any increase in activity will increase load and the level of increase will vary in a manner directly proportionate to load demand. The skeleton must also remodel to withstand the traction forces exerted by working muscle. At base level activity these forces are relatively small. However, as muscles build in response to increased demand, the traction forces rise sharply.

As previously stated, tissues respond and build as a result of the stresses to which they are subjected (Wolff's Law) and it is this rebuilding of the bone incorporated into the early stages of training that takes time, because bone is slow to rearrange and remodel its internal architecture. During the early stages of training it has been demonstrated that there is an initial de-mineralisation followed by a re-mineralisation. This research on a group of young horses (two, three and four year-olds from Texas A and M University) has also demonstrated that the mineral loss occurs during the first 60 days of training. The bone mineral content then appears to remain low for approximately a further six weeks, gradually returning to that considered appropriate for a continuation and increase of training requirements. This time span would match the training protocol of past times when at least three months of slow steady work was considered necessary prior to the commencement of serious training.

Periosteum

Bones are covered by a vascular membrane called the periosteum. As the bone remodels, the periosteum is often required to stretch. If the bone remodels too fast the periosteum may not be able to accommodate sufficiently. This situation gives rise to severe pain and in man this state is termed a 'shin splint'.

It is often periostial pain which is first felt by the horse before full blown sore shins, when minute stress lines visible on an X-ray develop. The stressed bone area, usually on the front of either the hind or fore limb cannon bones, may 'bulge' during the repair process, even remaining as a permanent feature. American terminology has been borrowed to describe this state as 'shin buck' or 'bucked shins'.

Training programmes

Work in man demonstrates that muscle activity achieves bone remodelling responses, hence the requirement for osteoportic patients to indulge in controlled periods of physical activity. However, there are no comparable stresses experienced by the human skeleton when compared with those encountered by the equine frame. The levels of force generated as the entire body mass of the horse lands on a single limb, after the suspension phase during gallop or when landing after jumping, are almost impossible to comprehend. Many trainers are returning to long, slow, distance types of preparation, interspersed with short sharp bursts of intense activity, these intense activity sessions introduced as the animal's general muscle tone improves.

Another factor to be addressed during early preparation is the consideration of the surface on which the horse trains. If a horse is always worked on a sand surface it will adapt to the demands of that surface. Obviously working on grass or on roads creates different demands. It must be a source of concern to all competitors if the surfaces encountered at competition change radically, for example jumping from turf and landing on a road, even if the tarmac has been covered in sand, peat moss or wood chips. The difference in compaction forces must take its toll, particularly if the animal's tissues have never been subjected to those types of stress. Thus it can be seen that a variety of surfaces need to be incorporated into training, as does the use of undulating terrain, this last to ensure that every muscle group exerts a traction force. Just going round and round in an arena does not activate the full muscle complement because, even though early training may be aimed primarily at bone remodelling, exercise is a multi-factorial affair.

As exercise demands increase so should mineral supplementation be considered, for to build the bones successfully the necessary components must be available or the stressed structure will borrow minerals from a site not considered to be under as much stress as that requiring remodelling. This inevitably causes weakness in the structure from which the ingredients have been borrowed.

As the number of horses suffering skeletal breakdown continues to rise, riders and trainers need to appreciate that training the skeleton is of paramount importance. They should implement an exercise regime lasting for at least 12 weeks, including activities arranged to promote gradual bone remodelling. This is achieved by using controlled concussive forces, road work and various muscle activities (such as exercise over undulating terrain). As the animals become conditioned, short periods of sharp work designed to increase cardiovascular competence can be added. It cannot be stressed too strongly that probably the most important factor in any training programme, be it for horses or humans, is to appreciate the necessity to allow sufficient time for the skeleton to adapt to training and exercise requirements.

It has been shown that excessive repetition of a single exercise is unnecessary, and that exposure to a wide variety of exercises for short periods of time is preferable during the remodelling phase.

A point often overlooked when considering impacts on the skeleton is the effect of shoes. A steel shoe will create a different shock to the aluminium plate. No human athlete would compete in a pair of shoes bought the day before a competition, nor would they change the angle of their foot to the ground, as occurs if the shape of a horse's foot is changed by shortening the toe for example. Obviously if a horse pulls a shoe it must be replaced, but surely it makes sense to reshoe three to five days before competition? Particularly if shoeing is long overdue, it is essential for tissue function to implement a regular shoeing programme and to make any necessary changes to foot shape slowly.

Muscles achieve movement in many ways: some convert the appropriate parts of the skeleton into levers, others stabilise body areas in order to allow the leverage system to propel the mass both in the desired direction and at the appropriate speed. Those muscles concerned with stability lie closest to the skeletal frame, their fibres tending to be short and arranged in patterns to allow 'give' rather than a large movement range. These muscles are called *postural muscles* and are the muscles prone to most damage when an area of the body frame is moved through a range of motion greater than it was designed to perform.

Muscles are arranged in layers, their shape, position and bulk creating the body's contours. When the muscles are conditioned, as they should be in all top athletes, those lying just under the skin are clearly visible. The individual muscle and bone landmarks visible under the skin is known as *surface anatomy*. Never forget mass is not muscle, many horses today carry far too much cover and they are assumed, because of their visible bulk, to be fit and are asked to perform tasks with unprepared muscles that are quite unable to sustain the effort required. Have you ever seen a very fat athlete? Weight lifters, cross channel swimmers and discus throwers are bulky but their muscle shapes are clearly defined. Sprinters and high jumpers are lean, while rugby players have well-defined, bulky muscles because they need stamina as do long distance and endurance horses whose shape differs from a flat race horse.

There is a distinct difference between a lean fit horse and a thin sick horse.

The muscles concerned with movement are composed of long, thin fibres, often from several origins and fusing into a single structure at their insertion. This format is designed for strength. Many are named appropriately: the *quadriceps* (quadra = four) is a muscle composed of four sections joining together to form the patella tendon in both man and horse. The whole complex structure is responsible for extending the knee in man and the stifle in the horse.

Training tissue involves many complex cellular interactions and, because cells have memories, mistakes are costly. Slow advancement, working to a logical programme, may take time but will lead to improved performance and reduce the risk of injury.

Chapter 6
Understanding Exercise

It needs to be understood that muscle tissue, be it in man or horse, requires preparation to achieve anticipated goals. It is almost impossible to write in a manner that achieves a multi-dimensional picture for the reader. Muscle is not flat, nor is it a single tissue. Within it lie nerves, blood vessels and lymphatic vessels, along with many varied cell types. All these components are involved in muscle function, so it follows that all these components will be required to adapt as muscle is prepared for increased activity.

No muscle ever acts in isolation, therefore any activity is described as 'group action'. All muscle activity is under neural (nerve) control. Before any sort of muscular training is initiated it must be remembered that gravity provides a constant force influencing the musculo-skeletal system. This influence is of sufficient importance to ensure that, even in an untrained subject, the muscle competence of each living animal will resist the forces of gravity exerted upon that individual.

The adaptation of muscle to cope with increased demand is very slow and perhaps the previous section indicates the complexities involved. Before considering total body training for either man or horse it is necessary to consider some of the terminology associated with muscle activity and the implications of different activities. Only by doing so is it possible to plan programmes for improved performance, and to use intelligently the many books discussing exercise, albeit mostly written in regard to human activities, where for a considerable time it has been appreciated that differing activities require specialist training protocols.

Muscle types

Prime mover (agonist) The muscle which initiates the first activity leading to a chain of events.

Antagonist Works in opposition to the prime mover, lengthening if the prime mover shortens or, shortening if the prime mover lengthens, ensuring a smooth movement.

Secondary agonist   A muscle group which may need to work to assist the prime mover if the task demanded is too great for one group of muscles.

Secondary antagonist   The muscle works against the secondary agonist ensuring smooth movement.

Stabiliser or fixator   Groups of muscles acting to form a stable, temporarily immobile area affording the prime mover an anchorage for the movement needed.

Synergist   Muscles working in harmony with all interacting groups during movement and ensuring economy by eliminating unnecessary, or excessive, activity.

Muscle work

Concentric muscle work   The muscle tissue shortens to effect the movement. Efficient and economic.

Eccentric muscle work   The tissue lengthens to effect the movement. This type of muscle work is very demanding and, if muscle is unprepared for tasks necessitating eccentric work, injuries are common. Downhill work demands eccentric muscle work, if you want to know what your horse feels like when performing this type of work run down a steep hill or walk down a mountain, your calves and thighs are working eccentrically. Register, unless you are superfit, the pain, not only that experienced at the time but also felt the following day.

Static muscle work   Muscles must 'hold a position', neither shortening, lengthening nor relaxing. Dressage demands a great deal of static work as the animal 'holds an outline'. It is the most exhausting of all types of work because the tension created during the work reduces the cleansing of the muscle and also the delivery of much needed fuel.

Range of motion

Movement of the body occurs when muscles move bone levers, and bones move one upon another at their connecting joints. The range of movement possible is dependent upon the anatomical shape of the joints as well as the flexibility of the soft tissues passing over the joints. The combination of these two factors controls the amount of movement that can occur between the bones forming a joint. The full range of movement possible at any joint is termed the ROM (range of movement) of the joint.

As a joint moves through its range of motion, all the structures that service the area are affected, the joint surfaces, joint capsule, ligaments, blood vessels, nerves, the lymphatic system and, of course, the muscles themselves.

Movement is usually described using terminology applicable to joints: flexion – bending, extension – straightening, adduction – adding to the body, abduction – taking away from the body, rotation – turning.

Muscle range is related to the functional activity of the joint or joints over which an individual muscle passes. Muscle range is taken to be the distance from complete elongation of the muscle to maximal shortening of the muscle. A simple example is to consider the human elbow. When the arm is straight, the biceps or 'bending' muscle is fully elongated, and if measured using a protractor the full stretch measured at the actual elbow joint would be 180°. As the muscle shortens it flexes (bends) the elbow. Then, due to both the construction of the elbow joint and the fact that the muscle bulk of both upper and lower arm meet, the 'bending' muscle is fully shortened (contracted) some 15–20° off the complete range described on a protractor.

Range of movement is broken down still further and the full 'arc' subdivided into:

- Inner range
- Middle range
- Outer range

Each range places a differing load upon the working muscle, and once this fact is appreciated it becomes possible when planning training to vary the work requirement by changing the range of movement at joints.

Inner range

Inner range is described as being the work achieved for the last 35° of movement; very little power is required or generated.

Middle range

Considered to be the arc of movement from approximately 145° to 45°. Work in this range is an excellent way to improve muscle capability.

Outer range

The arc of movement described as being from 180° to 145°. This range is economic at speed as the elastic recoil from the ligaments around the joint, stretched during activity, aids the movement.

Muscle composition

The actual composition of muscle fibre is still being investigated but in both man and horse three types have been isolated and described: slow twitch, fast twitch I and fast twitch II. There appears to be a genetically inherited predominance of fibre type. The flat horse has been selectively bred for speed over a short distance. Obviously speed is multifactorial, but to change the discipline of an animal bred and trained to go very fast over a short distance to another discipline, perhaps to dressage, takes years not months. Some breeds have a predominance of slow twitch fibres in their muscles and are therefore more suited to be trained for tasks that require stamina. The crossing of the Shire to the thoroughbred is an attempt to achieve a mix of the speed of the TB coupled with the endurance of the Shire. Before purchase it is always worthwhile, however much you like the animal in question, to stand back and decide what you want to do with the horse. The old proverb 'you cannot make a silk purse out of a sow's ear' is pertinent.

Slow twitch

These types of muscles have a complex but very efficient energy utilisation necessitating oxygen. As the name implies not only do they contract fractionally slower than fast twitch muscle but they are also capable of prolonged periods of activity. They can be considered as endurance fibres. The long distance runner and the endurance horse require a predominance of this fibre type and, despite the fact that all muscles are a mix, training methods can be adjusted to involve the recruitment of a greater percentage of the fibre type best suited to the task.

Fast twitch

Fast twitch fibres enjoy a slightly different chemical fuel base which allows very rapid energy conversion, this resulting in a greater speed of contraction. However fast twitch activity is only efficient for a very short period, the waste by-products eventually impeding muscle function.

To understand this muscle mix, it is essential to remember the requirement of both man and horse in their wild states. The wild horse recruited fast twitch fibres in an explosive burst of energy, enabling it to run away from its predators. It then reduced its speed and moved at a much slower pace as it continued to move away from the danger zone. Man recruited fast twitch fibres as he chased his prey and then recruited slow twitch as he either returned with his prize or walked sadly home.

Muscle function

Muscle must enjoy a nerve supply, and muscle tissue is incapable of functioning in the absence of a communicating nerve. When muscle activity is commanded by the brain in response either to a learned programme or to some external or internal stimulus, the nerve endings in the muscles recruited release chemicals to activate muscle firing. The recruitment is selective, occurring in units or sections. Each section is known as a *motor unit*.

Selection occurs in an orderly fashion and rarely is an entire muscle recruited. The number of motor units required are set to work and, as they become fatigued, other groups within the muscle take over in an imperceptible manner, allowing the tired units to cleanse and refuel. There is still much to learn and new concepts will continue to be developed in the light of increasing knowledge within the field of muscle physiology, particularly with regard to equine muscle.

The precise chemical interaction which causes muscle filaments to contract is not pertinent to this text necessitating, as it does, the understanding of complex chemical formulae. However it should be appreciated that the main muscle fuels are derived from fats and carbohydrates, not as many people seem to imagine from proteins.

Muscles are coordinated by the nervous system. Electrical impulses travel from the brain down the spinal cord. At every junction between the bones of the vertebral column that encloses the spinal cord a pair of nerves are formed. These thread-like branches move out into the body mass where they meet other nerves to form larger and more efficient branches. These branches in turn sub divide to supply the muscles. The sub dividing is in a manner that ensures *agonist* and *antagonist* muscle groups receive messages from the same main nerve, ensuring instant communication to both groups of muscle.

Fuel delivery

To achieve muscle activity the chemical energy in muscle tissue converts into mechanical energy. This chemical energy can be described as fuel. Some fuel is stored in muscle tissue. Training improves storage capacity, but that which is not stored locally must be delivered along with oxygen. The efficiency of this fuel and oxygen delivery is in turn dependent upon the efficiency of the heart which pumps the blood around the body.

As described previously, the capillaries form a network that invades all the tissues of the body. In order to obtain oxygen, the capillaries of the lungs embrace the air sacs (alveoli), enmeshing them in a 3D 'spider web' construction. Oxygen molecules move through the walls of the alveoli and into the capillaries, responding to a difference of pressures across the respiratory membrane. The pressure in the capillaries on the outer walls of the alveoli sacs is less than that within the sacs themselves. This pressure difference causes the oxygen molecules to migrate outward to the capillaries to equalise the pressure difference. As the molecules move into the capillaries they are attracted to red blood cells, and in healthy people and horses four oxygen molecules attach to each red blood cell for transportation to a selected site.

Carbon dioxide molecules return to the lungs attached to a red blood cell that has given up its oxygen molecules. The cells move first through capillaries then into veins to be returned to the capillary network of the lungs. Once there migration of the carbon dioxide into the alveoli sacs occurs in response to a pressure variation, but in reverse to that utilised by the oxygen molecules. Once in the alveoli sacs the carbon dioxide molecules collect and are expelled as unwanted gas.

This process of diffusion and uptake occurs for every blood-borne substance. The mechanism enables the collection of nutrients from the gut, essential ingredients from the liver and recycled waste from the kidneys, to name but a few processes of collection and delivery by the arterial blood. The venous blood carrying waste products delivers them to the appropriate organs that are concerned with waste excretion.

Blood moves around the body due to pressure within the arteries, and this pressure is achieved by the pumping action of the heart. The heart is a muscle and, in common with all other muscles, requires fuel and training enabling it to utilise its muscular walls to greater effect. As the muscle, particularly that area associated with the left ventricle, achieves greater efficiency so at each heart beat a larger volume of blood is expelled. This adaptation should also result in a reduced heart rate (number of beats per minute) and will almost certainly, in healthy subjects with all other systems working efficiently, reduce the time the heart takes to return to a resting normal following an exercise-induced increase in heart rate. This recovery time is a useful indicator of the fitness level of the subject.

The heart of the average horse weighs approximately 12 lbs, and some famous horses have been shown to have exceptionally large hearts. One, Secretariat, an outstanding thoroughbred from the USA, was discovered at autopsy to have a heart almost double the size of a normal horse. Therefore at each beat his heart was able to pump out at least twice the volume of fuel carrying blood enjoyed by others against whom he was racing.

The human athlete is able to monitor heart performance while training by using a heart monitor. This methodology has not been as successful in predicting performance fitness levels in the horse although a number of devices have been tried. Man is also able to monitor blood pressure, another useful health and fitness indicator not available for the horse.

The fuel demands of working muscle vary widely: muscle at slower paces may demand more fuel than muscle working very fast for a short period. However, fast paces over long distances increase demand; for example, in a horse at gallop the oxygen and fuel consumption in muscle is increased by between 70 and 100 times above resting levels.

As previously stated, the delivery of oxygen followed by waste collection occurs in tiny vessels, the capillaries. It has been calculated that between 4000 and 5000 capillaries deliver to and remove waste from each square millimetre of muscle under athletic stress. In order for this exchange to occur the blood is obviously not under the same pressure within the capillaries as it is in the arteries. As the waste collects within the veins the pressure exerted by the working muscles compresses the veins, squeezing the venous blood back towards the heart. All veins are equipped with non-return valves to ensure that the waste-laden blood will only move back toward the heart, thence to be pumped for reloading before once again setting out as arterial blood on the lengthy delivery round.

Following strenuous activity (which causes considerable production of waste) the complete removal of the waste will not have occurred by the time activity ceases. Studies conducted on human athletes following marathons demonstrate that full recovery can take several days. From the few studies on horses available it has become apparent that, while animals might appear normal on the day following competition, neither glycogen (fuel) reserves nor electrolyte balance are fully restored.

As the removal of waste is dependent upon uptake into the venous circulation and venous flow is assisted by the muscles squeezing the blood back to the heart, the old adage 'walk the last mile home' is explained. The long, steady walk, necessitating minimal muscle effort and therefore minimal fuel wastage but achieving compression followed by a period of relaxation, influences the venous system and aids the removal of waste. As a rider you should walk beside your horse for at least the last quarter mile. Swedish massage has a similar effect in aiding venous blood flow, although considerable skill is required to achieve sufficient compression in the huge muscles of the equine hindquarter. At competition most experienced grooms understand the benefits of walking their charges. Many have learned to massage, and there is now a small group of qualified masseurs trained to work on both horses and their riders.

Neuromuscular co-ordination

While the capillary network of the vascular system effects nutrient delivery and waste removal so the tentacles of the nervous system invade every body structure to co-ordinate, command and control every single body activity, both those under conscious control and those which occur automatically.

The nervous system is divided into two: the central nervous system and the peripheral nervous system.

Central nervous system

The central nervous system is composed of the brain and its extension, the spinal cord, which is the section lying within the canal formed by the bones of the vertebral column (backbone). The brain acts as a computer, analysing all incoming information, deciding upon the appropriate response and dispatching signals to achieve the response required. This is often a multi-signal delivery as more than one tissue type may be involved.

Magnified and in cross section the spinal cord resembles a main telephone cable. Multitudinous fibres are arranged in bundles or tracts, each tract having its own specific communication function. All commands from the brain to the body, and the responses from all body components to the brain, travel up or down one or other of the many tracts within the spinal cord. It is important to understand that, while in man considerable research and subsequent identification of the individual spinal tracts has been undertaken, this is not the case in the horse. Equine neuro-anatomy is poorly described in all textbooks and it should not be assumed until proven that the neuro-anatomy of man and horse are identical. For example, acupuncture is concerned with neural stimulation, but the 'point' charts for man and horse are not identical. To show the possibility of these differences we now consider the pyramidal and extrapyramidal tracts.

Pyramidal tract

This is related directly to the capacity of an animal to learn and execute highly skilled movements. Described by De Lahunta as being 'poorly developed in the horse, ox and sheep, in the horse there is a sizeable contribution to the facial muscles suggesting that these muscles perform the most highly skilled activity of the species'. The tract is highly developed in the human and is concerned with skills and fine movements of the hand. This is a major difference between the species.

Extrapyramidal tract

It is related directly to muscular activity required to support the body mass against gravity. It initiates voluntary muscle activity, controls motor activity, and controls muscle activity associated with respiration, cardiovascular function and most visceral muscle function.

While damage to any part of the central nervous system is not really pertinent to a text that discusses how to improve athletic ability, athletes do occasionally sustain injuries to the *central nervous system*. The tissue of this system *never recovers from serious injury*, thus an accident which destroys central nervous tissue will, dependent upon the area in which the injury is sustained, render that area incapable of ever again performing its allocated functions. A person who severs the spinal cord loses all movement and sensation below the area of damage. They are paralysed. If damage occurs within the brain itself the functions commanded by the damaged area cease to occur.

In man damage in the neck (cervical spine) creates a *quadraplegic* subject in whom all four limbs are affected. Damage to the mid or lower back affects the legs and the subject is a *paraplegic*. Spinal damage in the horse results in incoordination and the horse is termed a 'wobbler'. Brain damage may kill, cause fits, adverse behaviour or incoordination, depending on the site of damage.

Peripheral nervous system

The peripheral nervous system describes the nerves found within the body mass. These nerves originate from the spinal cord and are given off in pairs, one to the right and one to the left of the body, emerging through gaps between the vertebrae of the spine. The following shows the number of pairs of nerves emerging from different areas of the spine in man and horse.

	Cervical (neck)	Thoracic (chest)	Lumbar (loins)	Sacral
Man	7 pairs	12 pairs	5 pairs	5 pairs
Horse	7 pairs	18 pairs	6 or 7 pairs	5 pairs

Motor nerves are a sub division of the system. They deliver messages to command muscular function, the messages passing outward into the body mass. A sensory nerve reports back from the body mass to the brain. No muscle ever works alone. Agonist and antagonist muscle groups receive commands from the same nerves so that the groups work as a unit. *Training enhances neural ability.*

As the nerve enters a muscle it moves into the tissue and forms the *motor end plate*, at approximately the area where the middle portion of the muscle ends and the distal or final one third is said to begin. This motor end plate is a chemical command centre. Chemicals released at the motor end plate bind to chemicals already present within muscle tissue, and the combination of the two chemicals creates an electrical charge. This in turn triggers the chain reaction which allows the muscle tissue to convert its chemical energy into mechanical energy. Improved performance therefore depends not just on exercising the muscles to make them stronger, but also on improving by careful training an improved, efficient neuromuscular response.

Because the muscles are coordinated in pairs (an agonist with an antagonist), it is important that complementary muscle groups are exercised equally. The late James Hunt was instrumental in providing a set of gymnastic apparatus, the *Nautilus equipment*, which necessitated equal effort for both bending and straightening during activity. Swimming offers equal resistance to movement but does not build over-ground muscles in either man or horse. However, it is an excellent cardiovascular activity. The wearing of a weight also offers balanced resistance or loading during activity. When planning a training programme these factors should be considered, for example, if a horse is going to have to compete carrying 12 stone, training should be planned in a manner where the weight is gradually increased until the horse is able to easily carry 12 stone. At this stage the weight could be increased further so that when the time to compete arrives the actual weight of the rider is less than the weight carried during training, so the athlete will have plenty of reserve ability.

Neural input prepares the tissues, establishes sufficient reserves of fuel, and finely tunes the chain reactions required for muscular movement.

Fatigue

Fatigue is applicable to horse and rider and can be local or general.

Local fatigue

A muscle suffering fatigue responds by a reduction in capability. The onset of local fatigue may be due to one of a number of factors

- A decrease in energy stores
- Insufficient oxygen
- A build up of lactic acid
- Inhibitory commands from the nervous system
- Insufficient or inappropriate training

Muscle fatigue is associated with local discomfort and a decline in contractile ability. Man is able to recognise and report the symptoms to his trainer, but the horse will continue to try to perform as requested by its rider by recruiting other less tired muscles. This is usually uneconomical and American research suggests that micro trauma may occur as long as ninety days before manifesting clinically. If a horse repeatedly pulls up stiff or is suddenly unable to work as previously *look for a reason*. It is a great mistake to hope the problem will 'go away'. Often, massage or two or three sessions of exercises designed to target the area of discomfort will solve the problem and prevent the establishment of inappropriate uneconomical movement patterns.

General fatigue

This is the diminished response of the subject to perform to previous standards of even low intensity exercise, despite being allowed a normal recovery period. The reasons for general fatigue require extensive investigation:

- Is nutrition adequate?
- Is there an allergy related to food?
- Are the haemoglobin levels within normal limits?
- Is there a problem with oxygen uptake?
- Is the body temperature reading above normal limits?
- Are the electrolyte requirements being addressed?
- Is the subject suffering from a systemic attack (such as a viral infection)?
- Has the subject been overtrained or overworked beyond capacity?

In both horse and man specific blood tests can help to identify problems. The blood picture could be described as the 'barometer' of health. In man specialist blood tests have been developed to calculate bone health, primarily used to detect osteoporosis (loss of bone density). These *bone markers* have been replicated in equine blood as have *tendon markers*. These methods, when generally available, will be a valuable asset to trainers, particularly those training young animals. Both TB animals and those of mixed breeds (TB × Shire, for example) show widely diverse skeletal maturation. Warm bloods and ponies are also slow to develop.

Exercise-induced muscle soreness

Exercise-induced muscle soreness should not be confused with fatigue. The former occurs after unaccustomed activity or vigorous exertion, for example, if the subject which normally trains on good surfaces and in good conditions is suddenly confronted with deep mud, a strong head wind or high humidity. The discomfort and temporary stiffness will usually resolve within a few hours, provided adequate oxygen is restored to the tissues and circulatory flow is stimulated. The problem can often be avoided provided a period of 'cool down' is incorporated into the immediate post activity period. Once again, *walking the last mile home* has proven to be beneficial.

Training

Nobody becomes a competent athletic equine trainer overnight but there has to be a starting point. The aim should perhaps be to improve the physique and ability of each horse and rider to achieve a harmonious interaction between both.

One must aim to train the muscles to achieve the basic movement required and then to train the movements to achieve the overall function. In order to do this it is necessary to address:

- Strength
- Stamina
- Suppleness
- Skills
- Speed
- Specificity
- Mental attitude

The complexities associated with muscle training were really not addressed until the 1990s. In 1992 Sahrmann pronounced that faulty movement could induce pathology leading to trauma and that musculoskeletal pain syndromes were seldom caused by isolated events but were the consequence of habitual imbalances within the movement system.

Faulty movement

Incorrect movement patterns can arise from many things:

- Habit.
- Incorrect imprinting with the foal and the head collar (see page 45).
- An inability of the rider to command the horse correctly, resulting in

imperceptible changes of function, and incorrect movements in the horse leading to imperceptible changes in rider balance, causing trauma to both.

- Abnormal movements such as those that occur if the animal slips or the rider meets the horse wrong at some pace, in particular over a jump. Many people have stated that they felt their back 'go' as the horse landed.
- Faulty posture as a result of sub clinical pain.
- Tissue breakdown or 'pathology'.

One of the arts of both training the horse from the ground and training the horse when ridden is to be able to identify and immediately correct any dysfunctional or incorrect movement pattern before it is logged in the movement centre of the brain and becomes regarded as normal. It is important to be able to recognise and assess the interrelationship between the joints, the muscles and the nerves, because the nerves not only command the muscles but also lay down patterns of movement in the cortex. As we discussed earlier the horse has a brain adapted to record movement patterns and incorrect patterns are rapidly adopted. It is the re-establishment of normal, economical patterns to allow economical and non-traumatic movement that is one of the arts of training. It also follows that early training must be very specific in order to ensure that the movement patterns laid down in the brain of both horse and rider are those which will be efficient.

When training you are aiming to create a biological adaptation to improve performance in specific tasks. The type of response and adaptation will depend on the training methods adopted:

- Training the heart and the lungs (the cardio-pulmonary system) is essential for increased stamina.
- Muscle must be trained in order to improve performance.
- Training the nervous system is essential to ensure the correct response.

Improving muscle performance necessitates increasing the force against which the muscle must work – this is termed *increasing the resistance or loading*. Loading does not necessarily increase the size of a muscle and certainly does not do so in early training. It should be appreciated that overbuilding muscle in the horse may be detrimental because the equine skeleton is less able, because of its evolutionary mechanisms and makeup, to withstand the tremendous stress caused by over-strong muscle. During training, muscle that is loaded beyond its metabolic capability recruits dormant motor units present within its tissue matrix, for it appears that muscle has many motor units in reserve. There have been suggestions made that muscle strength or competence may also be increased in a manner which causes an increase in the number of muscle fibres, this increase caused by possible longitudinal fibre splitting. In laboratory animals this fibre splitting has been observed when the muscle groups have been subjected to very heavy resistance over a period of time. However, the findings have been difficult to replicate in the human and, as laboratory animals bear little resemblance to the horse, it would be unreasonable to presuppose that this is what occurs.

Increasing the competence of muscle puts extra demand upon all other structures, for example, the tendons, ligaments and bone. As the skeletal tissue becomes stronger and adapts to the increasing demands adaptation also occurs within tendons, ligaments and at muscular tendonous junctions. This last area is where muscle tissue changes its texture type, becoming more compact and changing to become tendon tissue. These adaptations take time and it is essential that they occur before excessive training begins. Increasing demands should be included in an exercise programme. Once again the absolute necessity for a long, slow and varied pre-training regime is apparent.

Exercise regimes

As with so many features in life today there are a serious number of misconceptions associated with exercise. There is a warped visual image of the health centre or home gym requiring us to spend time pumping iron, fighting machines until breathless, sweating and pink, not only in the face but also in the arms and legs. *This is not necessary, and not even useful.* Horses spend hours doing flat work, sweating and miserable. Far too many routines have been designed by people with insufficient knowledge of the requirements associated with physical activity. Even those who should know seem to get it wrong: the doctor who started the jogging craze, Mr Fix, in the USA, gave himself a coronary thrombosis, the very thing he was trying to avoid. The people who survive *do things slowly.* A survey of aspiring astronauts showed those who cycled to work each day demonstrated a higher level of general fitness when tested than those who pumped iron in a gym. A similar result was observed in a group of National Hunt jockeys. The regular golfers performed better when tested than the intermittent gym enthusiasts. A recent report regarding a community in the New Forest in the UK hit the press. The local GP had persuaded people to walk or cycle to the shop, and to leave their cars at home unless going on very long journeys. The local health record has improved to such a degree that other general practitioners are trying to persuade their patients that regular controlled exercise is the answer.

General considerations

To ride, certain areas of the body require consideration and the starting point before rushing off to classes needs to be a series of questions.

- What do you, the individual, wish to achieve both for yourself and your horse?
- Which areas of the body are important to target in order to improve or maintain present riding standards for you and your horse?
- Does one need strength to ride?
- How strong does the horse need to be?

Back to basics – the place of *Homo sapiens* in the hierarchy of the world is that of hunter-gatherer and that of the horse is as a prey animal with no conceived tasks other than survival. Species evolution is not in tune with twentieth century living demands. Natural man is geared to daily activity, moving over rough terrain to achieve balance, suppleness, stamina and endurance. The horse evolved to gently wander in a herd. How fortunate we are that we are all endowed with these primitive skills.

To ride you need:

- To be able to balance
- To be supple
- You require stamina, *not* strength

There is a difference, the long distance runner develops stamina, the weight lifter strength. Supple, pliable muscles are far more useful to both rider and horse than strong, bulky muscles. Stamina should be considered as the ability to perform repetitive movements over prolonged periods of time with only small changes of position. This is exactly what occurs in all riding disciplines, with the possible exceptions of show jumping and flat racing (in both competition time is short but both necessitate balance and stamina).

Balance ability requires mobility. Planning a riding programme, just as planning for any other sport, necessitates that the exercise and stretches incorporated should mimic the desired function of the appropriate body areas. Riding, unlike nearly every other sport, demands that both sides of the body work in unison. Training muscle coordination, joint movement and balance necessitate motor learning and neural adaptations. Many standard exercises performed in the gym are inappropriate as they work one side of the body, and then the other, rather than both at once. Step exercises are an example. There is no need to spend hours of specially allocated time in a gym exercising and stretching because it is perfectly possible and far more desirable to build the necessary exercise activities into daily life.

The necessity to train muscle in both man and horse requires knowledge of the various methods which can be implemented to load muscle and so improve performance. However, due to the important part played by the joints, essential to muscle activity, it is the joints which need early consideration. In man it is impossible to have a mobile ankle if the foot is stiff, similarly stiff ankles lead to stiff knees and so on, joint by joint up the body. In the horse stiff joints also create problems by changing the manner in which the shock waves generated at ground impact are distributed and absorbed.

Consider the implications in man, stiff fingers equals stiff wrists, elbows, shoulders, this stiffness not due to lack of muscle capability but caused by the reduced range of movement caused by impaired proprioceptive function. Proprioceptors are neural message stations. If a joint loses movement, poor quality messages result. The body is very economical, and reduced or loss of neural input results in reduced muscle function. Why waste energy servicing areas if they do not appear to be working and from where incomplete messages are being received? Perhaps an easy visual picture is to recall seeing a leg, one that has been in plaster after a bone fracture. When the plaster comes off the leg has 'wasted'. This means it has lost muscle. The muscle loss is not due to the break in the bone but to the inability of the joints within the plaster to move. The nerves which pick up signals caused by the joint and muscle movement are the proprioceptors. The knowledge regarding proprioceptive input has been relatively recently described and has led to the development in human medicine of a CPM (continuous passive motion) machine. People with, for example, a broken thigh bone, are strapped to a machine, after the break has been pinned or put in plaster, which moves the joints above and below the break. This stimulates the proprioceptors and muscle loss is nearly totally eliminated.

Horses with joint problems may also exhibit substantial muscle loss. For example, although all four feet are on the ground, careful note of the angle between the pastern and the ground will show when the weight is not being distributed evenly through all four limbs. The pastern of the limb carrying more weight inclines at a more acute angle to the ground, while the pastern of the limb with least weight will be nearly vertical. The weight is not being distributed through the limb containing a painful joint. Horses also may demonstrate loss of bone density in the affected limb, particularly if the imbalance of weight has continued for a long time

Stretching

Because stretching to increase joint range affects other local structures, it is best done with the feet on the ground. This is not possible when stretching equine limbs and so the very greatest care should be taken when stretching activities are attempted. If a stretch is performed in a weight-bearing situation the safety mechanisms with which the body is endowed activate to *avoid* over-stretching. These mechanisms do not operate effectively in a non weight-bearing situation, and so non weight-bearing stretches often lead to minor injury. It cannot be emphasised enough that great care should be taken when manually trying to stretch both equine and human joints.

It is difficult to persuade a horse to stretch but it is perfectly possible by working it in long reins over poles. The distance between the poles is increased so the animal must increase stride length, stretching all the working structures in a balanced manner in each of the four limb levers. Some horses will stretch on their own, putting both forelimbs out in front of their body and bending down in the manner of horses trained in the circus to bow to an audience.

Equine flexibility is just as important as rider flexibility, as is joint range, but the latter is also associated with conformation. For example the horse with a very straight shoulder will never be capable of a very long stride, a person with deep hip sockets will have less movement than someone with shallow sockets. Any form of stretching needs to be performed when the subject is warm, and no stretches should need to be performed more than 3–5 times at any one session. The effect of stretching will not be instantaneous, it will take 3–5 weeks to achieve an increase in flexibility of the structures around the joints. To over-stretch in an attempt to achieve marked improvement in one session is detrimental, causing micro-damage to the tissue architecture with consequent scarring and permanent loss of mobility.

Unfortunately many stretching exercises advised are described without the feet of the subject in contact with the ground. The body expects to have foot-to-ground contact. The soles of the feet in all species are richly endowed with neural sensors, not only for balance, but also to initiate the body's own safety mechanisms. Consider these facts when choosing stretch techniques – if it is necessary to lose foot-to-ground contact ensure the stretches performed are within the normal range for the body part being stretched.

Improving muscle

In order to improve muscle capability it is necessary to increase the workload and this can be achieved in a number of ways by using resistance.

Resistance

Resistance is present when any dynamic or static muscle contraction is opposed by an applied force. This force can be applied:

- Manually
- Mechanically
- By positioning the body in order to lengthen a working lever (limb)
- Utilising the subject's own body weight against gravity

Concentric

Concentric relates to muscles working as they shorten against a resistance. Sit-ups in the human achieves concentric abdominal work and concentric hip flexor work. In the horse most normal work demands concentric activity, and an effort increase can be achieved by choosing an appropriate range of muscle activity.

Eccentric

Eccentric relates to muscles working as they lengthen against a resistance. If a human lies on his back with knees bent and then straightens the knees so that the legs are at an angle of approximately 45° to the ground, he will first do concentric work using the thigh (quadriceps) muscles until the legs are straight. As the straight legs are lowered to the ground the abdominal and hip flexor muscles are used working eccentrically. In the horse down hill work requires eccentric muscle activity, but the paces must be controlled. The horse will try to create an easy pace and this will not achieve the object of the planned activity.

Isokinetic

This term refers to movements that occur at a constant speed. Because the speed of the limb movement is constant the resistance which these types of exercises provides will not vary provided the range of motion remains constant. For this reason isokinetic exercises are sometimes referred to as accommodating resistance exercises. In the human this type of exercise can be carried out using light weights that are moved repetitively and at a constant speed. In the horse work at a constant repetitive speeds using a resistance, such as an incline either up or down, will produce this type of exercise. *It has been shown that isokinetic exercise is a very effective means of increasing muscle power and endurance.*

Isometric

This form of exercise is a static exercise. A muscle must contract or work without any appreciable change in length and without any visible joint motion. Although little physical work is achieved, the tension creates changes in muscle.

This type of exercise is particularly useful for the rider who needs to work muscles in a static manner, but at the same time maintain suppleness in the upper body, head and neck. Adoptive changes in the muscle begin to occur if the isometric contraction is held for a minimum of six seconds. This time period allows for peak tension to develop and for the necessary metabolic changes to begin to occur within the muscle.

A good way to achieve this in the upper body, head and neck is to press back against a chair back when sitting down. This type of muscle work occurs in the horse when certain restraint gadgets are used. Care must be exercised when applying restraint to ensure that the muscles appropriate for the eventual task are being influenced.

Closed chain

Closed chain exercises refer to movements that occur when the body moves over a fixed segment. In the human, for example, the foot is planted on the ground and the body is lowered to a squat and then returns to the vertical.

Closed chain exercises should be performed with some degree of weight bearing in the positions that are going to be adopted in the eventual sport. Because closed chain exercises are performed in weight bearing situations they stimulate many of the nerves sited around joints. Therefore, besides improving muscle strength and endurance they also improve balance, coordination and functional agility.

Sitting on a child's space hopper and bouncing achieves a closed chain activity (see Fig. 3.2). A horse worked down a long grid with identical spacing between every pole achieves closed chain activity. Closed chain exercises are probably the most useful for all riders.

Chapter 7
Considerations for Rider Preparation

Twentieth century living has radically changed the lifestyle of many people. The general health of individuals suffers by being exposed to adverse levels of a vast array of pollutants and also, due to ease of travel, exposure to a host of micro-organisms. These are naturally present and cause no problem to persons in whom resistance is present, but cause havoc in others lacking an indigenous immunity, a scenario similar to that occurring when Captain Cook took measles to the South Pacific and all the inhabitants of Easter Island perished.

To exercise in order to achieve an improved level of general fitness requires responsible consideration of personal health goals. A general health check, before rushing into a complex fitness programme, is only sensible. Most GPs are happy to arrange a blood test and, just as in the horse, it can indicate your health status so that any obvious problems can be addressed. Just as in the horse, the condition of hair, skin, nails (hoofs) are also indicative of metabolic excellence or deficiency.

Nearly every health club and public gym have trained instructors who are there to help people by testing their level of physical fitness and suggesting a routine appropriate to each individual. The rate of the heart is calculated first at rest, then following activity on a static bicycle, a step machine or treadmill. This will indicate, by the time taken for the resting rate to re-establish, the efficiency of the heart. The efficiency of lung function is also closely linked to heart rate recovery.

Muscles cannot increase their efficiency in the absence of fuel and oxygen, and in this respect, you, the rider, are no different from your horse.

Just as in the horse vitamins and minerals are not stored against need. It has been calculated that at least 94% of the contents of all the mineral and vitamin supplements taken are excreted, so overdosing is all too common. Minerals and vitamins have the same functional roles in both horse and man (p. 50).

Riding is different from every other athletic activity and, as in all sports, there are specific areas to be considered.

Rider target areas

Feet

The muscles on the sole of the foot work in partnership with the ankle. Stiff feet equals stiff ankles and vice versa. The bones and soft tissues of the human foot are designed to form three spring arches. As the body weight passes down through the foot into the ground these arches collapse, then, as the body weight passes forward to be transferred to the other foot, the arches reform, utilising a spring-like recoil built into their soft tissue structures. The foot was stretched as a result of the downward weight bearing compressive factor, and the energy for recoil derived from the stretch of the soft tissues. It is a very economical design.

Ankles

The ankle is controlled by groups of muscles: the calf muscle at the back of the lower limb, the *gastrocnemeus*, ending in the Achilles tendon. Down the front of the lower leg and slightly to the outer side are the muscles that work in partnership with gastrocnemeus muscles, the *anterior tibial muscles*. These balance the activities of the calf muscle.

A third group lying on the outer side between the gastrocnemeus and the anterior tibials are a group named the *peronei*. This group is very important to the rider as they move the heel and foot when the knee is bent, taking the fore foot outward or laterally then stabilising it so that the 'aids' can be administered through heel or spur contact.

Knees

The knees of the rider need to be 'bouncy' as they are working when riding in a manner that is described as 'unlocked'. This unlocking is secondary to the fact that when a person is seated on a horse bareback or in a saddle the hips externally rotate. The knees are controlled by the thigh muscles, those on the front known as the *quadriceps*, those at the back known as the *hamstrings*. The knee is designed to flex (bend) and extend (straighten) but not to twist (rotate). However, when bent, the muscles can achieve a twist of the lower part of the limb on the upper, this movement occurring at the knee. Similarly the muscles around the hip can rotate (twist) the upper body on the bent knee. The knee joint itself has no muscles primarily designed to perform these rotation movements. If the twist (rotation) is excessive the internal structures of the knee joint, the cartilages (menisci) and/or the internal ligaments, the cruciate ligaments may be damaged as both these sets of structures are designed to prevent, rather than allow rotation.

The hip

The hip joint is the strongest joint in the human body, its internal stability and strength ensured by the *ligamentum teres*, a structure within the joint running from the hip socket on the pelvis to the ball-like head of the femur or thigh bone. The ball and socket construction allows for multi-axial movement but, just as in all other joints, the structure is dependent upon its musculature to initiate and control movement, both the range of movement and direction. The joint is perfectly capable of positioning itself to allow the rider to sit astride but the relative position of the head of the thigh bone (femoral head) to the socket is foreign to the hip joints. The joints do not naturally and easily allow the relaxation required within the muscle group that runs from the inner side of the upper thigh to pubic bone (base) of the pelvis. These muscles are named the *adductor group* because they stabilise the leg toward the central mass. They also create the front 'arch' of the rider's seat (p. 36).

The buttock muscles extend the leg on the body and are also important in preventing the upper body being pulled toward the ground by gravity if the subject leans forward. They are programmed for this activity when weight passes through the hip joints. In the saddle rider weight is redistributed from the joints to the muscles and the two bony prominences in the buttocks so balance must be relearned. A new proprioceptive reflex needs to be established. Lifting the leg upwards when lying face down works the buttock muscles.

Lower back

Too much emphasis is placed on the *mobility* of the lower back or lumbar spine. All movement starts from a fixed point and the lower back needs to be *stable* not *mobile*. Attempts are made to strengthen the lower back with emphasis on the abdominal muscles. Their function is to bridge the gap between the bottom of the chest cage and the upper brim of the pelvis, creating a container for the abdominal contents. The fibre construction of the muscles is designed for minimal excursion. Back extension exercises work the muscles which run from the shoulders to the upper portion of the lower back at which point they 'marry' into a fascial sheet. Therefore the normal lifting of head and neck does not involve active muscle activity in the lumbar area. Similarly, lifting the leg upward when lying face down works the buttock muscles.

The lower back is stabilised by groups of muscles attached to the bones of the spine. They are in pairs, one on either side of the centre line of the bones. Inside the pelvic cavity are the *ileo psoas* muscles (fillet steak, if you enjoy meat). The loin area of all animals contains these muscles. The second set of muscles are found at the back of the bones forming the lower back area, the *multifidi*. These sets of muscles work together to stabilise the area, coordinating with the intervertebral discs, in shock absorption.

Mid back

The mid back is designed to support the ribs and allow some rotation. The cage formed by the ribs is a semi-rigid structure containing the lungs and heart. Its ability to expand to increase respiratory ability is crucial for oxygen uptake. Some of the new body protectors are very unyielding and seriously impair the necessary excursion of the chest wall.

Shoulders and arms

The shoulder complex, called the *shoulder girdle*, resembles a milkmaid's yoke. The shoulder blades (scapulae) are attached to the back of the chest wall and join the collar bone (clavicle) just above the shoulder joint. The collar bones continue forward to attach to the breast bone (sternum), so completing the yoke.

The arms hang from below the outer ends of the yoke. The whole complex relies on muscles for attachment to the body frame. The only connecting joint is the very small one formed between the sternum and collar bones. The muscles are arranged in a manner that allows the arms plenty of movement at their junction with the yoke, but also attaches the whole complex to the body frame in a manner designed for strength rather than a large movement range. The muscles lying across the front of the chest, *the pectorals*, can become too strong so that they easily overcome their antagonist group at the back, the *rhomboids*. This pulls the shoulder yoke forward reducing both respiratory capacity and arm and shoulder efficiency.

Neck and head

The construction of the neck allows considerable movement in every direction, the least mobile segment being the junction between neck and chest. The head is balanced on two shallow, saucer-shaped indentations on the upper surface of the first neck bone and a small bone peg projects upward from the second, the design ensuring stability. The muscles work to both hold the head in a balanced position and to allow freedom of movement. This is a complex requirement, necessitating layer upon layer of minute muscles. It is for this reason that neck injuries take so long to recover.

It is essential to ensure that protective head gear really fits. Some type of fall is inevitable for all riders. National Hunt jockeys fall, on average, once in every seven rides and riding horses carries a risk which is why it is sensible to achieve an understanding of the body preparation required to make certain you protect yourself correctly and bounce easily.

Gymless rider preparation

Few riders have time to spend in a gym to try to get fit to ride, so is a gym essential? No, it is perfectly possible and preferable to incorporate useful exercise activities into daily life. When possible, exercise both sides of the body simultaneously. Remember, this is preparation for a sport where the body must learn bilateral activity; a one-sided rider will always experience problems.

Feet

Mobilise the feet in the bath. It is much easier to activate and exercise the tiny muscles of the feet in water and also when they are visible.

Toe activity: Curl and stretch the toes open and close the toes and move them in sequence.
Mid foot activity: Turn the soles of the feet in toward each other, then turn the soles of the feet outward.
Medial and lateral arches: Put both feet firmly against the end of the bath. Imagine you are trying to pull the balls of the feet toward the heel, this raises both the medial and lateral arches, leaving toes and heels in normal contact.
Transverse arch: With the feet still in contact with the bath end raise the area just behind the second, third and fourth toes, this exercises the muscles of the transverse arch. If this is difficult resist the area with the tips of two fingers and push the foot upwards against the finger pressure.

Foot mobility is essential for total body mobility. The soles of the feet are endowed with myriad sensors programmed to prepare all the body components to adapt to activity in order to avoid injury.

In the bath all these activities employ concentric muscle work. When standing, the medial arch is assisted by a ligament, the *spring ligament*. If the exercises are repeated in standing, the raising of the arches employs concentric muscle activity, lowering them employs eccentric muscles. The most useful piece of furniture for rider preparation at home is a four legged kitchen/dining chair.

Ankles *(Fig. 7.1)*

Isometric exercises: Sit on the front half of the chair. Place the inner side of the heels against the outer side of the two front legs of the chair. Keep the knees apart using clenched fists, side by side. Press the heels inward against the resistance afforded by the chair legs and hold for 10 seconds. Release. Repeat 10 times. Rest 30 seconds.

Place the outer sides of the heels against the inner side of the two front legs of the chair. Press outward against the resistance afforded by the chair legs and hold for 10 seconds. Release. Repeat 10 times. Rest 30 seconds. As the muscles begin to improve alternate each set, inside then outside, and repeat three to five times.

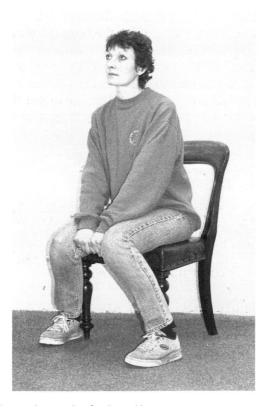

Fig. 7.1 Isometric muscle exercise for the ankles.

Hips and limbs

Hip adductor muscles (isometric): By squeezing the clenched fists between the knees the hip adductors have performed isometric work during the ankle routine.

Hip abduction (isometric) and shoulder adduction (isometric): Place the clenched fists one on the outer side of each knee. Push inward with the fists and resist the pressure with the legs. Hold 10 seconds then release. Repeat 10 times. Rest 30 seconds. Repeat the set three to five times.

Hip flexion (isometric), chest muscles (pectorals, isometric) and arms (static): Place the hands, palms down, on the tops of the knees. Press down with the hands and press up with the knees. Hold 10 seconds then release. Repeat 10 times. Rest 30 seconds. Repeat the set three to five times.

Hip extensors (isometric): Relax the arms and push down into the chair seat with the buttocks and thighs. Hold 10 seconds then release. Repeat 10 times. Rest 30 seconds. Repeat the 'set' three to five times.

Active muscle work lower limbs (concentric, eccentric): Hold the arms as if holding reins. Position the feet with the toes below the bent knees, knees apart as if in the saddle, and lift the buttocks off the chair seat by approximately nine inches. Hold for 10 seconds. Sit down slowly. Repeat 10 times. Relax 30 seconds. Gradually increase the number of sets. This exercise is much more difficult than it sounds. Note that it is possible to do this exercise off-balance. It is important that the weight is evenly distributed on both legs, and the hands are in the correct position.

The lower back

Stabilisation for the lower back (concentric and eccentric) (Fig. 7.2): Stand in comfortable balance, keeping ankle and knee fixed. Lift the straight leg from the waist until the foot is approximately two inches off the ground and hold for 10 seconds. Replace the foot and lift the other leg. Hold for 10 seconds. Alternate the legs, lifting each 10 times.

This is an easy exercise to perform during daily life, when cleaning teeth, answering the telephone, standing at the sink or cleaning tack. To feel the muscles working stand with the thumbs pressed against the back just below waist level, one on either side of the spine. Perform the exercise and it is possible to feel a hard 'cord' form on the side of the lifted leg. If the area feels 'soft' you have a weak lower back. This activity builds the ileo psoas (fillet steak!) and the multifidi.

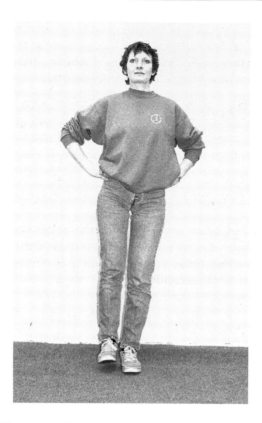

Fig. 7.2   The hip hike to strengthen the muscles of the lower back.

It takes a minimum of six weeks to build these muscles. Exercise on the hour every hour to be successful in rebuilding your back.

To prove the muscles perform a different function during walking leave the thumbs on the back and walk. It is impossible to feel the muscles.

Mid back and neck (isometric): When sitting in a high backed chair press your back against the chair (the chair must be tall enough to resist the back of the head). Push back and hold for 10 seconds, then release. Repeat 10 times. Rest 30 seconds. Repeat three sets.

Do not do this exercise when driving, unless the car is stationary.

Other good exercises

Mobilising the shoulders, upper back and neck: Hold a towel diagonally across the back, one hand at waist level the other above the opposite shoulder. Pull the towel up and down for 10 to 15 seconds. Change the diagonal and repeat as before.

Massage the lower back and mobilise the hips: Hold the towel at waist level and below, one hand on either side of the body approximately six to nine inches from the body sides. Hold the towel taut and move the lower body and buttocks from side to side for 10 to 15 seconds.

Cardiovascular exercise (closed chain balance reflex): Beg, borrow or buy a child's space hopper or medicine ball. Squat, gripping the ball between the knees and bounce until breathless. Rest until heart rate and respiration return to normal, then repeat.

Hip/leg stretches (Fig. 7.3): Flexibility in the adductor group of muscles is essential for all riders, and tears or damage in this group is catastrophic for any rider.

Stand astride feet facing forward. Keep the upper body upright. Move the upper body sideways until the knee towards which the body moves is bent. The opposite leg should register a feeling of stretch inside the thigh. Hold the position for 10 seconds.

Swing the body in the opposite direction, at full stretch balance and hold the position for 10 seconds. Repeat 10 times for a set, then rest for 30 seconds. Repeat three to five sets.

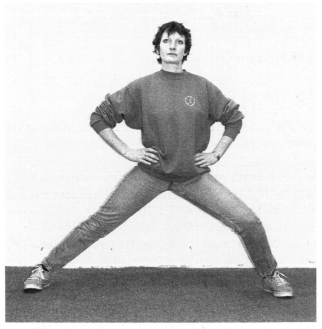

Fig. 7.3 The adductor stretch for the hips and legs. A wide stance is necessary to perform this exercise correctly. Keeping the body upright, swing the body slowly from side to side until a feeling of stretch is experienced on the inner side of the straight leg.

Improving muscle tone: Muscles are programmed to function, not in isolation, but in conjunction with the entire body during activity. Muscles increase their power and endurance capabilities when resistance or loading during activity is increased. The wearing of aerobic weights during normal daily activities improves muscle capability (Fig. 7.4). One on each wrist increases the loading for all upper body activities. One on each ankle increases the loading for all lower limb activities.

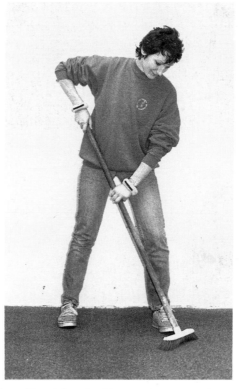

Fig. 7.4 The use of aerobic wristbands while performing everyday tasks to strengthen the muscles of the arms and shoulders. Weights are also available for the ankles.

Practising rising to the trot for balance (Fig. 7.5): From a chair, practice rising to the trot, aiming to maintain your weight evenly on both legs, and keeping your hands in the correct position.

(a)

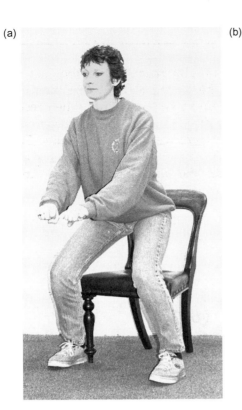

(b)

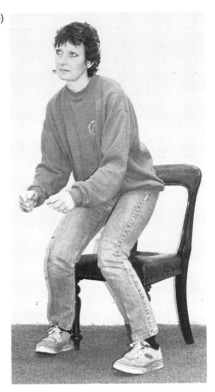

(c)

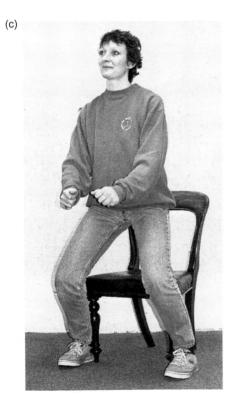

Fig. 7.5 Practising rising to the trot. (a) The weight is evenly distributed but the hands are incorrect. (b) The rider's hands are improved but she is now off balance. (c) The hands are nearly in the correct position and the balance is improving.

Practising how to feel the correct pelvic angle (Fig. 7.6): Fig. 7.6(a) shows the orientation of the bones of the pelvis and hip. Fig. 7.6 (b–e) shows how the angle of the body can be altered to affect the position of the pelvis in the saddle.

This approach is more effective for riders than hours in a gym where muscles are targeted selectively and therefore dependent upon the apparatus selected and programme chosen. No programmes have been designed for riders in the same manner as for other sports, where the appropriate muscle groups and coordinated patterns have been addressed in relation to the eventual requirements of the sport.

Cycling: Cycling recruits the lower limb muscles and can also be used as a cardiovascular exercise. It is an activity based on diagonals but improves muscle tone and increases endurance capability. Riding standing on the pedals, without using the saddle, increases the resistance substantially.

Running or jogging: Improves general body tone, and with the incorporation of hills improves cardiovascular efficiency.

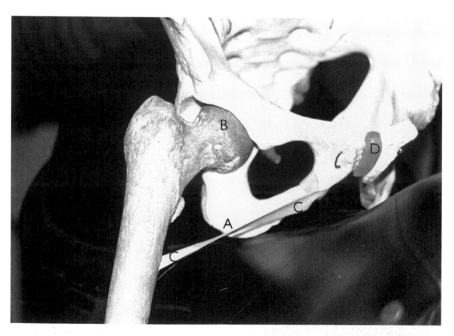

Fig. 7.6   (a) The pelvis viewed from the right side. The pelvis and hip are positioned correctly in the saddle. A – ischial tuberosity (seat bone); B – hip joint in slight external rotation; C – position of the adductor muscles; D – symphis pubis. Saddles are shaped to avoid putting much weight on this area, to prevent discomfort. People who have bruised the junction between the two parts of the pelvis can hardly walk.

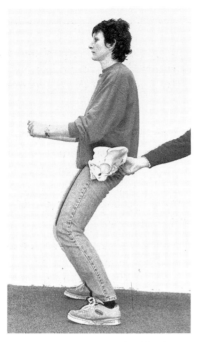 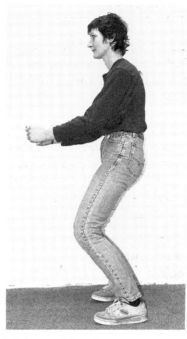

(b) Pelvis at the correct angle, allowing good balance for hacking and flat work.

(c) Balance achieved.

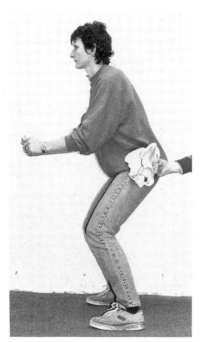 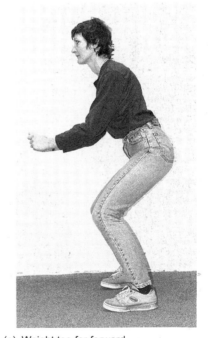

(d) Pelvis tipped too far forward. This causes the rider to have a very hollow lower back.

(e) Weight too far forward.

Fig. 7.6 *Contd*

Skipping: Useful as a total body activity, and lower limbs, ankles and feet especially benefit. Riders should jump off both feet.

Swimming: Improves muscle tone due to the resistance afforded by the water. Can be used to stimulate cardiovascular activity. *Do not* swim breast stroke with a weak back. The stroke creates a 'hinge' action in the low back, increasing the risk of further injury.

Many people will feel the activities suggested are inadequate and that they must punish their bodies in a gym. The choice must be that of each individual, but remember, riding and being ridden requires *suppleness*, *balance* and *bounce*, not just strength. Muscle bulk does not benefit either horse or rider.

Chapter 8
Considerations for Equine Preparation

Mechanical objects created by man are rapidly and continually updated. Consider computers. We are living in a world where the norm is instant fix and throw away rather than save, conserve and recycle. Horses are not machines with replaceable parts, they are a miracle of chemical interactions and biomechanical engineering.

Preparation for athletic demands in the horse requires a long, low, steady preparation. There is no instant fix, there are no training aids, special rugs, specialised gadgets, coat shines, special diets, special bandages or therapies which will change a naturally ordained order of progression developed over millions of years to produce an equine athlete. The equine athlete, even in a natural state, is capable without training to produce a performance which would equal that of a human runner moving at around 45 mph, and to keep up that speed over a considerable distance. (The zebra, first cousin to the horse, can run for up to 100 miles to reach water when the rains come.) However, for the ridden horse, the sequence of events necessary to prepare to carry a rider and then to compete require consideration of the basic principles utilised by any human athlete.

Points to address

- General health
- Diet
- Skeletal preparation
- Joint flexibility
- Cardio-pulmonary training
- Adequate exposure to the experiences required at competition
- Progressive muscle loading (discussed in the following chapter)

General health

It is impossible to train a horse that is not well. The animal cannot describe if it feels well or ill so it is essential to learn to 'read' each animal. There are many health pointers and all need daily consideration, for the onset of an illness occurs often for no known reason and the horse may be well one day and ill the next.

Stockmen read their stock and it is only possible to learn to do this by constant observation. Books can tell you what to look for but the art of husbandry is a continual learning curve. Look and observe day in day out until the observations become habit and it is possible to recognise and record changes without thinking. Note the condition of coat, mane and tail, eye brightness, gum colour, hoof growth, the smell, colour and amount of urine produced, and the colour and texture of the droppings (faeces).

50 years ago, no doctor ever examined a patient without looking at their nails (hoofs), hair (mane and tail), eyes, both for brightness and the colour of the lower lid, and questions regarding urine and faeces (droppings) were also routine. Nothing has changed, you need to learn to read the condition of your horse by constant observation.

Feet

Hoof growth is, just like human nails, a major health indicator and the condition of the hooves is critical for performance. It is the hoof which is the first body part to make ground contact at all gaits. It is the weight-bearing base of each limb, its shape determines the angle of the joints and limb bones to the ground. The bulbs of the equine heels are loaded with sensors, constantly recording and communicating with the motor areas of the brain and the centres concerned with balance. Foot fall, limb sequence, muscle coordination, gravitational balance and adjustment to uneven terrain are some of the many requirements that need sensory input from the feet.

The frog

The frog contracts and expands as a pressure pump, aiding the return of venous blood from foot to body mass. A dry frog, a diseased frog, susceptible as it is to fungal invasion such as thrush, cannot work efficiently and the entire body suffers.

The sole

The sole of the foot should be slightly moist as it too moves during ground impaction. The hoof is not a totally rigid structure and it deforms and reshapes to aid the dissipation and absorption of all impaction forces. Just like all other body tissues the foot has its own nutritional requirements and these cannot be obtained by rubbing in preparations. If the necessary components are missing the foot will be dry, break easily and grow slowly, mimicking the manner in which the human nails behave if there is a nutritional deficiency or following illness.

Trimming

You should never try to save money by extending periods between either shoeing or regular trimming. Even horses turned out in the field bare-footed for their holiday must have regular foot attention. There is an old saying 'no foot, no horse' and a horse with poor quality feet will always have problems. The animal will be a poor quality athlete and also produce secondary joint problems as it endeavours to reduce the discomfort in its feet, doing so by landing incorrectly at the expense of the limb joints, particularly the fetlock joints (ankles).

Read the feet

The surface of the hoof sometimes exhibits ring-like bulges running around the outer wall surface from heel to heel. These rings may indicate a period of foot growth at a time when nutritional changes occurred. The condition of the hoof above the individual rings show if the change was good, indicated by a smooth oily texture, or poor, indicated by a dryish, rough texture.

Ask advice before using supplementation if you observe hoof wall changes. Balancing nutrition is not a 'hit and miss' affair. Ask your farrier, feet are his job. The laminitis centre near Wooton Basset in Wiltshire also run a help line.

Feet may be flared out on one side, and this is usually associated with unbalanced ground contact and incorrect break over. The causes may be conformational, imbalance of the foot, sub-clinical pain in the foot or limb, or habit, the latter often associated with a problem that has resolved. Always remember the horse rapidly adopts incorrect movement patterns if avoiding pain and retains those patterns until taught to re-establish the pre-pain patterns of movement.

A 'boxy' foot occurs when the horse reduces weight through that foot when standing.

A 'flat foot' occurs when most of the weight is taken through that foot when the horse is standing. These variations are most common in front feet, the horse often having a flat foot on one side, a boxy foot on the other.

Squared off toes are common in hind feet and one foot or both may be affected. The horse may be lazy, slopping along and making no effort to lift its hind feet. There may be sub-clinical pain in a limb joint of the affected hind leg or it may be a habit pattern established in response to past discomfort.

Under run heels. A long toe forces the body weight backward onto the heels which gradually collapse, changing the angle of foot to the ground. This is detrimental to the entire limb, changing joint angles and increasing tendon stress. Try pointing your toes upward taking all the weight on your heels, walk first and then try to run with your foot in this position. You will feel strain and discomfort in all your limb components.

Long toes and under run heels in a horse are a cause of more problems in joints, tendons and ligaments than almost any other condition. The condition, just as any other foot problem, takes time to rectify. To implement the changes necessary to reshape feet *cannot be achieved in one shoeing*. All the structures of the foot need to readjust, rearranging their internal architecture in response to the change of angulation.

Before asking your farrier for a change of foot shape consider the animal in question, its origins, breed and task. Flat thoroughbred horses from the USA have rather donkey-shaped feet when compared to the 'soup plate' shape of the original British thoroughbred. American horses need to dig into the dirt on which they race for stability. In the UK where racing is mainly on grass, the greater the surface area covered by the foot the less the animal sinks in.

European warm bloods imported to the UK for dressage have small feet and high heels. This is a breed characteristic in many and to try to give these animals a British foot shape is a disaster, often causing lameness. It may also drastically change the animal's performance for the worse.

Look at the feet of your horse and learn to read its health and way of going. Discuss problems with your farrier as they may be able to suggest a solution.

Coat

The hair comprises a part of the skin complex, the skin being the largest organ of the body. The individual hairs of the coat work in partnership with the sweat glands and both assist in temperature regulation. Each individual hair possesses its own minute muscle. As the animal becomes cold these muscles contract, raising the individual hairs in order to entrap air between them and create a layer of insulation. To the human eye the coat then looks as though it is fluffed up – have you ever seen a Shetland pony on a cold day?

If the coat is 'stary' (that is, it is not lying flat), feels rough to the touch, feels dry, or, when picked up, it and the underlying skin feel taut rather than slippery, one or more of these findings indicate that the animal is unwell rather than cold. In a healthy horse the coat should shimmer, shine, feel like silk to the touch and have a rapid elastic recoil.

In the heat, the hairs lie flat and no air is entrapped. The sweat glands excrete moisture which dampens the coat and therefore achieves heat loss by evaporation.

Show sheen and other similar concoctions which laminate individual hairs interfere with natural temperature regulation. Udder cream or other preparations liberally applied to limbs and belly prior to the cross country phase at three-day events do the same. The resultant insulation, created by creams or sprays, substantially reduces the area available for heat loss when temperatures are high. Daub if you wish to insulate (this is the method used by cross channel swimmers for insulation) but *not* if you wish to retain natural temperature control! The udder cream theory is that the horse will 'slip' over fences but this is very unlikely. After all, in the slippery pole competition the pole is greased, not the competitor's feet. This greasing has become accepted in the event scene although it was certainly not used in the early days of the sport.

Mane and tail

The texture of the horse's mane and tail vary, dependent on breed, that of the heavy horse being somewhat coarser than that of the thoroughbred or Arabian. Whatever the degree of coarseness, mane and tail should feel pliable to the touch, not too dry, and should brush out easily.

Gums

The colour of the gums should be pinkish, not white. Very white gums are usually an indication of a low haemoglobin level. At competition a failure for gums to return to pink, remaining white after finger pressure, usually indicates dehydration.

Eyes

The eyes should be bright with an alert expression. Pale lower lids and dull eyes indicate that all is not well.

Urine

The urine should not smell, it should be clear and not overly yellow in colour, it should be profuse, neither scanty nor cloudy, and passed as an easy, full flow, as though a tap is running, not dripping. Dark urine passed after competition usually indicates a state of dehydration. The dark colour may also occur following a rapid breakdown of energy components. It may also indicate that the animal has been asked to perform at a level too demanding for its current state of fitness or is not taking in sufficient liquid. Check that the water is not brackish and that the bucket is clean inside.

Droppings (faeces)

The droppings will change colour dependent upon diet. Those of the animal grazing are green, those of the stabled animal a brownish colour. The droppings should not smell and should appear as well formed, moist pellets. Hard, round pellets indicate dehydration, so food or hay should be dampened before being given.

Cow pat-type droppings indicate that the food has passed too quickly through the hind gut. These type of droppings need serious consideration as the hind gut is the area in which the main absorption of nutrients occurs.

The presence of whole food particles such as corn, oats or barley indicate a tooth problem. Primary grinding is not occurring properly and under these conditions digestion will be affected and nutrition will be inadequate.

You know how you feel before becoming unwell and you learn to read the indications. The horse feels much the same, but the only way that it can indicate any problems is through the medium of mood change, performance changes and body condition changes.

Your skill as its keeper is to learn to observe, recognise and act upon these signals.

Skeletal preparation

Early training should concentrate on conditioning the frame and strengthening the postural muscles. For this there is no substitute for long, slow, steady work which is undoubtedly the most important part of any training programme. The length of time spent in this phase will depend upon the age, previous activity of the animal and the time period since concentrated training or activity ceased. This preparation period, called by many LSD (Long Slow Distance) should incorporate walking, trotting and slow cantering. The tissues need an overall exposure to exercise to implement any adaptive changes.

Using the theories of Monty Roberts, it has been possible to achieve accelerated learning and improve obedience when breaking a horse to saddle and bridle or to harness for driving in a shorter time period than before, but even if your horse has been broken in the Monty Roberts way it will still require three to six months of steady, low-grade work to achieve skeletal stability. If the horse has been broken in the 'old fashioned' way, driven in long reins for 6–8 weeks, it will require approximately four months of steady, low-grade work to achieve skeletal stability. Any horse coming back into training after a holiday or change of discipline will require a minimum of six weeks, and preferably 12 weeks, of long, slow, steady work.

The muscles closest to the frame or skeleton are known as *postural muscles*. Quite simply it is their job to ensure the stability of the skeleton and to retain the anatomical positions of the bones comprising the frame, ensuring that the anatomical arrangement is neither over-stressed nor repositioned incorrectly as the animal begins to work.

During work, the bones experience stress caused by muscle pull and ground impaction forces. As all tissues remodel in response to the stresses they meet there will be a gradual change in both bone architecture and strength. Muscle responds relatively quickly to activity, but other structures (bones, joints, their attendant ligaments and tendons) are very slow to adapt to increased loading.

The skeleton of the horse takes approximately 25% longer than muscle to adapt to stress. Modern methods, incorporating as they do the early inclusion of interval training, appear to be creating problems and injury levels in competition animals having risen dramatically in the last decade. Riders, it seems, do not understand the necessity of giving their animals time in the early stages of preparation. The more strenuous the eventual task, the greater the preparation time needed to build the frame.

During this early work, exercise time is gradually increased from a brisk half hour walk until the animal is walking, trotting and cantering for up to two hours each day. Hills should be incorporated, as should work over uneven terrain. It is impossible to prepare a horse for competition in an arena because no animal can learn balance on a manicured, flat surface. Even dressage horses need variety. If the length of time taken for early preparation seems excessive consider the preparation of the human athlete, who certainly does not stand in his room for 23 hours out of every 24, exercise for an hour, and then compete.

Once the basic slow, steady work is complete, increased activity can begin. No matter what the animal's eventual discipline, nothing can beat the combined use of the exercises of the classical school and the use of cavaletti. The classical movements have been utilised down the centuries to:

- Build muscles, those of both posture and movement
- Initiate closed chain reflex responses
- Achieve suppleness and obedience

Many of the exercises can and should be executed with the horse in long reins. Surely it makes sense to teach, or re-educate, difficult muscle combinations without the added weight or possible confusion caused by a rider.

The use of cavaletti progressively loads working muscle and improves suppleness, as well as continuing to teach the discipline of activity. Cavaletti are the equine equivalent of human gymnastic apparatus. Riding over them is an excellent rider activity, improving balance and suppleness.

As the horse progresses it is also essential to improve cardio-pulmonary function. Asking for exertion at speed burns glycogen rapidly, putting the body into a state of oxygen depletion. Neural receptors are alerted and signals are generated commanding the heart to beat faster to deliver the much needed oxygen and, at the same time, breathing (respiratory) rate also increases. The heart is a muscle and, like all muscle tissue, responds to progressive loading by increased efficiency. As the efficiency of the heart improves, it is able to pump a greater volume of blood at each beat. The heart is then described as having improved its *stroke volume*. An increased volume of blood enhances oxygen collection and delivery. The oxygen debt reduces, and when the neural receptors signal an improvement, the heart rate slows, eventually returning to normal.

Unfortunately if the training stresses utilised during early training to improve bone density, muscle activity and cardio-pulmonary function are totally removed from the training schedule, after a remarkably short period of time the competence achieved by the training methods begins to be lost. It is therefore necessary to incorporate all the factors included in early training at least once every seven to ten days. This requirement is a relatively recent discovery and emphasises the need for a programme which, to many, must seem to include unnecessary retraining following a holiday or enforced lay off.

Joint flexibility

When planning a training programme you must always remember that the horse evolved as a running species which, over millions of years, has adapted to ensure speed for survival. The limb joints, while dependent upon flexibility, are governed by tendon extensibility for economic function. The front legs of the horse equate to the middle finger of the human hand, the back legs to the middle toe of the human foot. Because support is by tendon and ligament only (*no muscles are involved*) it must make logical sense to keep the load these digits will bear to minimum by keeping the horse light. Another feature sometimes not appreciated relates to the fact that the bones of joints do not 'lock' one into another, as do the pieces of a jigsaw, but are instead suspended by their soft tissue structures, muscle, tendons and ligaments. Imagine these as beautifully developed springs. Inadequate preparation of these structures leads to damaging compressive factors within joints and irreversible damage may occur. The hyaline cartilage in particular, coating the articular surfaces of all joints, is extremely thin in the equine and is not designed to accommodate the continuous concussive forces experienced by the modern horse as it works or competes. In the wild horse, these forces occurred for much shorter time periods and without rider weight.

Many horses are allowed to become far too fat and there is a *serious* misconception that an animal must be well-covered, looking rather like a prize bull, in order to be ready to compete. Unfortunately this notion tends to be perpetuated by judges on the show circuit and monstrous animals gyrate round the ring stressing every limb joint. Treatment is then required to control windgalls (wind puffs) and filling occurs in hocks and knees. Obesity in man is causing grave concern, creating as it does many health problems. The same applies to horses, and being overweight is particularly damaging to yearlings. Many are undoubtedly allowed to become grossly over topped, often during their sales preparation or for the show ring, where fat seems to mean fit. Surely discerning judges and prospective purchasers must realise how easy it is to mask conformation faults with over topping?

To save young joints and prepare them for the future the body mass must be adequately covered but not overly so. There should also be adequate space for movement and play at *all paces*. This really is very important, young animals should run out of energy and slow down by themselves rather than have to suddenly 'put on the brakes' by running up against a fence, so stressing knees, hocks and stifles. As feet determine joint angulation regular, balanced trimming is essential for joint development, as is a balanced diet containing adequate minerals.

Passive stretching for joint mobility

Passive stretching of individual limbs is discussed in all massage routines, but it is worth considering the normal range of movement of each joint and to work within that range. Always remember that when the foot loses contact with the ground some of the fail-safe mechanisms within the joints of that limb will *not* operate, thus it is possible to move a joint beyond its acceptable normal range and cause damage. The only joint in which it is impossible to achieve a full range of movement is the fetlock. The resistance afforded by the suspensory ligament, deep and superficial flexor tendons defies, as it should, any manual attempt at fetlock extension. Just as in the human athlete any attempt at manually improving joint flexibility should only be attempted after a suitable warm up.

The adage 'walk the first mile out' (just as 'walk the last mile home', mentioned on page 72) has a good reason. The athlete has been prepared and warmed up, all structures, including joints, ready to experience and cope safely with strenuous activity. Far too many animals from all disciplines are injured by being compelled to start working before being adequately warmed up.

It is not only the limb joints that require flexibility. It is essential in the neck joints and probably the tail, although little is known about the manner in which the tail aids balance, but it is certainly not there just to flick off flies. For example, the horse raises its tail to initiate a closed chain reflex which braces the hind legs just before it takes off to jump, and it also tucks its tail in to increase tension in the musculature of the croup and loins before bucking. A horse that clamps its tail while working will tend to have a stiff hind leg action, so clamping is an indication of discomfort in the croup or loin area. The animal clamps to ensure that muscle activity, which might cause pain through movement, is restricted to a minimum.

The horse's back requires to be stable rather than mobile. The construction of the equine vertebral column is such that, during activity, two sections are subjected to the greatest movement stress. These areas are located at the junction of neck to chest and at the junction of loins (lumbar vertebra 6) to pelvis. This last is in complete variance to man, in whom *stability* at the junction of low back (lumbar vertebra 5) to pelvis is essential. Mobility of the neck can be addressed by the use of a carrot offered between the front legs, or high in the air so the animal must stretch up (often left out), and on each flank, to achieve sideways movement. Gentle tail circling relaxes the hind quarters and back, and most horses seem to enjoy this method. Linda Tellington-Jones incorporates the technique in her routines with great success.

Cardio-pulmonary training

Without an efficient heart (cardio) and without adequate oxygen (pulmonary) there is no hope of athletic competence. The use of short or medium length bouts of intense activity, separated by short rest periods to allow partial recovery after intense activity, has been proven as a conditioning technique for the cardio-pulmonary systems of human athletes, and was used by Roger Bannister in the 1950s. It has been studied and refined by successive human athletic trainers and the method is now known as *interval training* or IT. The method has only relatively recently been applied to equine training.

The short periods of intense activity create metabolic demand in the working muscles and to service this requirement both heart and respiratory rates rise. The rest intervals are designed to achieve a partial, rather than a full resumption of normal heart and respiratory patterns. Before full recovery can occur, the next bout of activity begins, necessitating (as previously) increased oxygen uptake and delivery to service muscle demand. While involving the cardiovascular and pulmonary systems, the method is also aimed at conditioning muscle by stressing metabolism and energy conversion. This type of exercise is *not* designed to strengthen muscle, rather it increases muscle stamina by enabling muscle to accommodate the demands of increased activity.

It is often difficult to decide at which moment in an equine training programme to incorporate IT, for the limb structures must have been adequately prepared during the LSD phase to withstand the requirements of IT. Each horse, just as each human athlete, will require its own programme, the variables adjusted according to the final work load requirement. These variables are:

- The distance covered between each rest period ⎫
- The speed over the ground   ⎬ a 'bout' of activity
- The length of rest periods   ⎭
- The number of bouts of activity and rest incorporated to create a *set*
- The number of sets

Some horses do not take to IT, fussing or refusing to settle in the rest periods. In this case the Scandinavian approach, known as Fartlek (roughly translated to mean 'play at speed') can be utilised. Horses are worked slowly over longer distances, utilising the gait of their sport but the work is interspersed with short periods of high speed activity. To many this method may seem to create unreasonable exercise demands, but it does work well in developing a fit, healthy horse. For many the Fartlek method is easier to incorporate into a general training programme than IT, which necessitates a carefully calculated regime to be really effective.

Chapter 9
Progressive Muscle Loading I: The Addition of Resistance

Once skeletal preparation and stability has been achieved using LSD exercise, it becomes necessary to incorporate activities to increase muscle work load in order to continue to improve the capabilities of the muscular system. To achieve this necessitates the inclusion of a factor known as *resistance*. Resistance is achieved by progressively loading muscle, and to do so by designing activities that necessitate increased effort. The end effects are to improve:

- Muscle fibre recruitment
- Endurance capability
- Power
- Metabolism
- Capillary density
- Neural response

To increase resistance or load, it is necessary to plan a programme and to incorporate a variety of activities thereby creating a series of differing tasks. In human athletic terms this is known as creating a *circuit*. Just like the human athlete the horse should *not* be asked to repeat an exercise again and again and again. Variety is *essential*. Could you go into a gym and do press ups for an hour?

Equine apparatus

The apparatus available for the equine gym consists of poles, cavaletti and jumps. Programme design, to create loading, is achieved by informed choice from the options available:

- Classical exercises – long reins
- Classical exercises – ridden
- Ground poles – long reins at walk, trot and canter

110

- Raised poles – long reins at walk, trot and canter
- Small fences – long reins at trot and canter
- Ground poles – ridden at walk, trot and canter
- Raised poles – ridden at walk, trot and canter
- Small fences – ridden at trot and canter
- Grids (six or more cavaletti) – loose schooled, trot, canter
- Grids – ridden at trot and canter
- Changes of pace – transitions up and down
- Changes of direction – circles, serpentines

Progressive loading is achieved on open terrain from the following options:

- Grass slopes – lunge at walk, trot and canter
- Grass slopes – ridden at walk, trot and canter
- Road hills or grass – led off a second horse at walk
- Road hills or grass – ridden at walk or working trot
- Small fences – ridden on the flat
- Small combination fences – ridden on the flat
- Larger fences – loose schooled if possible
- Larger fences – ridden at trot and canter
- Fences on slopes – ridden at trot and canter up and *down* hill

All programmes should incorporate changes of speed, and also relaxation or rest periods. A horse finds it difficult to maintain a shape for lengthy periods in early training. It needs to stretch and relax before trying once again to respond to requirement. A slow progression ensures obedience, balance and muscle adaptation.

Circuit training

Circuit training incorporates controlled activity and ensures adaptive changes in muscle. The muscles, forced to work in a manner necessitating repetition at low intensity, demand oxygen to enable them to continue aerobic activity. After a period of time an increase in the density of the capillaries supplying the muscle fibres occurs. This is called *improved vascularisation* and improves the delivery of oxygen to the muscles. If long, slow activity is not included in the early training programme this improvement in vascularisation does not occur and so, during strenuous activity, oxygen requirement cannot be met. This leads to an excessive build up of both carbon dioxide and lactates, which may cause muscle damage leading to tissue breakdown.

When planning any training programme the choice of activities and exercises, both in the arena and in open terrain, needs to be made carefully to try to replicate the eventual functional demands the horse will encounter, or to improve the scope and capability of an animal already reasonably prepared but required to compete at a more advanced level. Fig. 9.1. shows an example of a circuit in an arena. The series of obstacles have been designed so that each demands a differing limb action, thus varying muscle activity. It is impossible to write an exact recipe because each horse is an individual and each will respond differently, both in the time required to learn and for muscles to condition. The circuit can be used to achieve:

- Muscle endurance
- Muscle strength
- Body balance
- Obedience

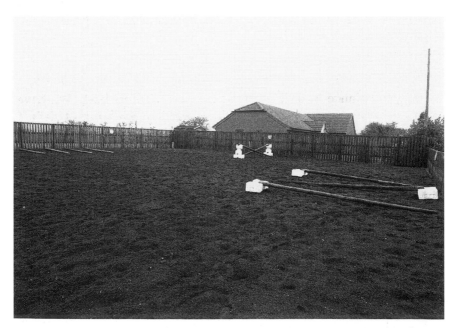

Fig. 9.1 The arena can be set up as a circuit with a variety of obstacles, each demanding a differing limb action to vary muscle activity.

Endurance

To develop endurance following improved vascularisation, active exercises need to be repeated over a prolonged period of time against a moderate load. Steady hill work achieves this. As we now know, muscle responds and builds to the loading it experiences. To increase loading walk straight up and straight down a hill and also work diagonally across a hill. These activities will work the muscles of the back, hindquarters and all the stabilising muscles of the limbs. Going uphill does not build muscle in the forelimbs as effectively as going down hill. The work that the forelimbs experience as the animal goes down hill is eccentric work and, as discussed earlier, this is one of the most exhausting and therefore the most stressful methods of loading muscle tissue.

Strength

Strength refers to the force of output generated in working muscle. Strength training requires muscle to work against a heavy load for a relatively low number of repetitions. In the horse the utilisation of the animal's body weight is the only method of increasing loading. Jumping down a grid of raised poles at all three paces (walk, trot and canter) creates the effort required to improve muscle strength and therefore the force of contractile ability. Using a weight cloth adds to the weight of the body mass, thus increasing load. Trotting and Hackney trainers use weighted boots to increase load.

Balance

Learning to balance in tack is a skill the horse has to learn. We have already seen that the horse can co-ordinate within a few hours of birth, it can balance after an hour or two and, should the foal miscalculate, it is free to recover unencumbered by any form of restraint. Problems for the horse begin as soon as breaking in commences, not just when the animal has to learn to carry man.

Tack is a restraint and it directs the manner in which the animal may move. Failure to move as the tack and manipulation of the tack by the trainer demands often results in pain, which leads to tension, and tension to anxiety. Each horse, just like each person, balances differently.

Working a horse from the ground and using side reins will begin to change the natural postural balance of the animal, a re-education necessitated by the alteration of the angle of the head and neck to the body. The rider will eventually communicate this requirement via reins and legs, as some flexion of the neck is necessary in order to lift the back to carry rider weight. Remember that this stage is very difficult for the young or inexperienced animal. Try to put yourself in the animal's place. Envisage a situation where restraint has hampered your movement. For example something as stupid as a three legged race. You are attached to another person whose movement and appreciation of movement is entirely different from your own. Only with skill and practice is it possible to coordinate.

The horse has first to learn to coordinate in a differing body position, that is the position demanded by tack, and then to learn to have rider weight added to its frame. No sooner has balance in tack been mastered then all its balance skills have to be relearned. The addition of a rider necessitates not only learning how to cope with an unstable weight but also how to coordinate new muscular activities. The groups of muscles adjacent to the backbone have to change function. Previously they were required to harmonise with and absorb tiny vibrations resulting from the forces generated as individual limbs met the ground, plus they resisted gravity. With a rider, the muscles must act to prevent the back from collapsing downward and at the same time assist in the maintenance of balance by counteracting any instability created by rider weight moving laterally outside the animal's centre of gravity. Obviously, if the rider is supple rather than stiff, skilful rather than apprehensive, secure rather than insecure, the horse will benefit. You can experience what it might feel like to be a horse with a rider on board by playing 'horsey' with a small child. Your back will soon tell you that it has had enough.

Horses raised on hills or mountain slopes have a better balance perception than those whose only experience has been on flat land. Balance perception is essential for both performance and safety. Activities to learn balance should be incorporated within general training. Cavaletti arranged as a fan, slopes, direction changes and working on uneven ground and jumping off angles all help. An old fashioned method of making a horse accustomed to carrying an unstable weight was to secure a bag of sand to the saddle or roller while working the animal from the ground. The horse had to learn to cope with the movements created by the weight before being ridden.

Obedience

Obedience is essential not only for performance but also for horse and rider (or trainer and groom) safety, and to avoid unnecessary injury. Obedience is not just compliance with rider command. It involves all general behaviour. Just like small children, foals should not be allowed to become domineering – they need to learn to accept restraint and to remain calm when handled, led or tied. Remember, lessons should be short, for a foal's attention span is similar to that of a small child. Two and three year old horses are the teenage group, exhibiting a 'try and see how far we dare go' attitude.

Early work in long reins is an excellent medium for discipline. It teaches acceptance of tack, the square halt, not turning in to the handler when on a circle, stopping when told, backing up, working over poles and cavaletti calmly, not rushing, refusing or ducking out. Horses should not be allowed to snatch when offered a treat or a carrot, bang the door when waiting to be fed or bite the people working with them. In the herd, bad behaviour is punished by the dominant mare, a swift reprimand soon teaching the necessary lesson. Very often a voice change from the handler, accompanied by one smart, light slap with the back of the hand on the neck achieves respect without fear or resentment. Continual half reprimands or the use of whip or broom do little other than create irritation, fear or anger, accompanied by loss of confidence and repeated incidents of bad behaviour.

Some readers may consider these suggestions unkind, but the horse handled sensibly will never be a threat. If allowed to become assertive it can lead to serious harm, not only to those handling it but also to other horses. A boxer's punch is of Lilliputian proportions when compared with the striking forces generated by the limb of a horse, neither does the boxer punch with steel knuckle dusters, probably the nearest equivalent to the horse's shoe.

Problems associated with training overload

Overload describes a state when an exercise progression has exceeded the current state of body adaptation. A useful method of detecting possible overload is by daily leg observation and palpation (feel). Fetlock filling, knee filling, hock filling, extra warmth, a slightly spongy texture in place of a firm one, early minor splint formation or tenderness, an early curb, all suggest that programme loading has been too demanding or insufficient time has been allowed for the body to accommodate. Go back one or two stages but do not stop the animal completely unless advised to do so by your vet.

Remember, it is better to vary, on a daily basis, all conditioning routines, thus minimising the risk of overload and fatigue by continuous repetition. RSI (repetitive strain injury) occurs as a result of repeated, similar overload activities.

Fatigue

In the human athlete, scientists in the USSR have demonstrated that the maximum number of repetitions for any single training activity in an exercise session should not exceed seven. Fatigue is complex and describes the diminished activity of muscle tissue in response to an activity stimulus. This diminished response is a multi-factorial problem. Amongst the many factors involved are a decrease in energy supply, a build-up of lactic acid, insufficient oxygen delivery, and an inadequate circulatory network.

Fatigue occurs if muscle has not been allowed time to adapt to a particular exercise, especially if the increase in the capillary bed has not occurred because early training has been hurried or omitted.

Damage to muscle as a result of fatigue is a serious problem. Motor units self-destruct and very often recovery occurs through scarring. This reduces the capability of the affected muscle group permanently.

Recovery from exercise

Adequate periods of time to allow recovery following exhaustive exercise sessions should be built in to every training programme. Muscle requires time to replenish the energy utilised during exhaustive exercise and to rebuild damaged tissue. Scientific studies show that light exercise, performed during recovery periods, enhances eventual recovery, thus the owner or rider should consider exercising the horse at an exhaustive level for three continuous days, followed by three to four days of light exercise to allow recovery.

Studies addressing equine recovery from North America and Australia suggest that on the day following competition the horse should be walked slowly for approximately one hour, or put on a horse walker twice for two half hour periods and also turned out for 2–3 hours, weather conditions permitting. On day two, the horse should be exercised at a brisk pace for up to one hour, combined with being turned out, weather conditions permitting. It appears that day three is the critical day for recovery and this is the day on which the horse should be allowed total rest. This means no ridden activity but, weather permitting, the horse should be turned out into a paddock. Training recommences on day four.

Up until recently, all concepts of muscle recovery have been taken from research on human athletes. The increased interest in equine sports physiology will show how applicable human-based theories are to the horse. Until this research is published there can be no hard and fast rules concerning fatigue and recovery but an intuitive owner or rider will read their horse and should be able to assess its level of fatigue recovery.

Turning out to aid recovery

Turning a horse out to grass is not unkind, every horse should be allowed the freedom to move, roll and graze unrestricted. Many paddocks are unfortunately over stocked with horses, resulting in the destruction of the pasture, particularly in wet weather. People lucky enough to own grazing will find their horses are healthier and easier to keep and handle if the animals spend several hours a day out in the paddock. Once the routine has been established horses do not gallop madly around when freed. New Zealand rugs are excellent for turning out and in cold or wet conditions the neck extension is essential. Field sheds are rarely used but are useful for haying in winter to avoid trampling.

The late Captain Tim Forster, the well known National Hunt trainer, trained many of his stars from the field, as do all the New Zealanders. It is normal procedure in New Zealand. It is amusing to note that when BHS examiners asked a trio of world-class event grooms what they did to their horses following International three-day events, Fiona (Blyth Tait), Jo (Vaughan Jefferies) and Penny (Mark Todd) all chorused, 'turn them out'. Apparently they nearly failed their exams, their approach considered negligent. Not so, it is natural.

The effect of gymnastic exercises on the muscular system

Lungeing, long reining and work in hand

Lungeing

Sadly, today's understanding of lungeing is to put on a bridle, often with no cavesson, with or without side reins, these attached if used from bit to roller or saddle. By the restraint of a single line, or rein fastened either to the bit or to the central ring of the cavesson, the horse is made to circle around the trainer. This method is of little or no benefit to the horse as it usually spins like a whirling dervish on the end of the lunge line. This is not lungeing. Unfortunately, the 'dervish' spin tends to be, not the exception, but the rule, particularly when the trainer is trying to lunge in a large arena, in a paddock, or, pre-competition, in an open area.

Lungeing is viable in a lungeing ring, where the outer perimeter of the circle is usually high-sided or boarded in. This enables the horse to be controlled within a circle of set parameters. The size of the lungeing ring varies but the average lunge line is 6 m (20 feet) in length. The animal should be encouraged to work on a large circle, for the imbalance achieved by an untutored or immature animal working on a small circle does more harm than good. Nearly all European lungeing methods employ both a handler and an assistant.

The activities concerned with lungeing are considered to be far more complicated than those concerned with long reining, for when lungeing the handler must keep the horse between lunge line and whip. He must ensure that no lateral head tilt occurs, that the hind limbs track in line with those of the forehand, and that perfect balance and cadence are maintained. If side reins are employed, care should be taken to make certain they are fitted in a manner that allows the natural outline of the horse to be retained until the animal has settled (Fig. 9.2).

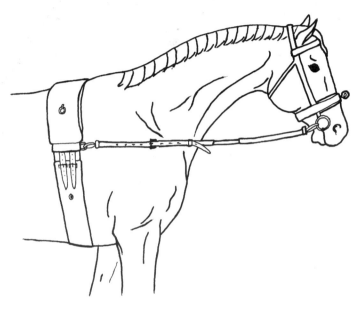

Fig. 9.2 Side reins. These are useful when the horse is being lunged or worked in long reins. They should never be used to impose a head carriage, and the horse should be allowed to balance itself with relying on the support afforded by side reins.

It should never be forgotten that, in early training, many experiences are new to the horse, no matter if the horse is being prepared from the ground or with a rider on its back. If a horse, taught to trot or canter from the ground, over bends and goes behind the bit, why should it change its way of going when ridden at trot and canter? It is essential to achieve from the ground that which will be required when riding commences because reprogramming is very difficult.

The reason that many of the European masters of equitation, both past and present, have built horses from the ground is to ensure that the musculature is fully prepared and each activity learned before the animal is asked to carry rider weight. To work a horse from the ground correctly when not in a lunge ring requires considerable practice. Fig. 9.3a shows a horse being worked correctly on the lunge. Far too many horses, even in a ring and correctly tacked up, are allowed to rush. 'Motor biking', they

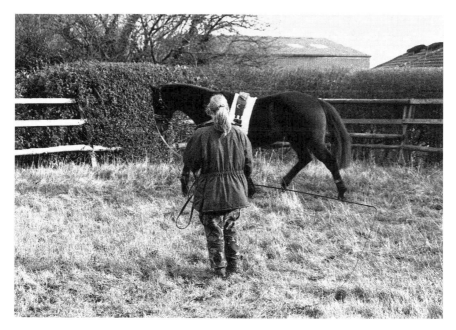

(a)

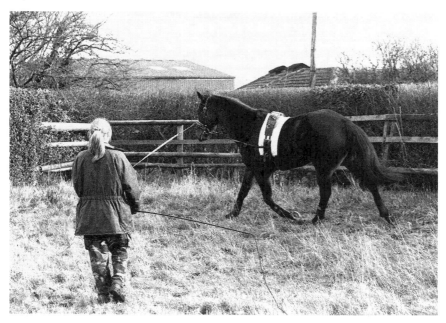

(b)

Fig. 9.3   (a) A horse working correctly on the lunge. Neither the side reins nor the line are being used as a prop. The horse is carrying itself and is working between the line and whip. (b) A horse on a lunge but off balance, falling in behind and using both the side reins and lunge line to lean on.

lean in, tracking incorrectly, the hind legs making their track away out-side that of the forelegs. This is not working or learning, it is just teaching bad habits. Whenever working, as discussed in the previous paragraph and in the section on imprinting earlier in the text, a horse learns to move in a way it has either adopted for comfort or has been made to use. A movement does not take long to become habitual but it takes a long time to unlearn the habit and to establish a new, advantageous set of move-ment parameters.

'Tying' the horse into a shape when first on the lunge achieves nothing, as the animal learns to lean, using whatever device has been utilised, to balance itself (Fig. 9.3b). The situation is similar to that of a child who has learned to ride a two wheel bike using stabilisers. Remove the stabilisers and they wobble and fall – balance must be relearnt, addressing the new situation.

Begin by letting the horse learn to balance without restraining aids, other than possibly a pair of loose side reins, and gradually introduce the restraint preferred to achieve the new position required. Most gadgets tend to create flexion only at the poll and this is not acceptable because the hind quarters merely 'tuck' and the animal trails the hind legs. Remem-ber, there are two ends and a middle to consider! This incorrect habit can be seen in horses who are working behind the bit with exaggerated flexion at the poll, their nose somewhere near the chest, showing active front limbs but little hock activity and with a hollow back.

When working from the ground be careful never to restrain the horse to such a degree that forward movement is constrained. It is preferable, unless you are an expert, to work off the cavesson rather than the bit. A roller is preferable to a saddle and adjustable side reins, partly elasticated, should run from the snaffle bit to the roller.

It is difficult for a novice, whether the novice be the trainer or the horse, to achieve work when lungeing. Remember, exercise is not work. It is very difficult, almost impossible, to achieve a perfectly balanced circle in an untutored animal if the trainer is not practiced in the art of using a lunge. As in any work programme, begin at a walk, progress to a trot and finally to a canter when balance and evenness of pace have been achieved. Try to work the horse by voice command in preference to flicking the lunge whip. The whip should be utilised for guiding, *not* for painful encour-agement or punishment.

Effects of lungeing

Correct work on the lunge builds the muscles of the back and loins, particularly the postural muscles (those closest to the back, named, as in the human, the *multifidi*). Although the equine back is designed to be loaded (the abdominal contents and gravity exerting a downward force which the vertebral column must resist), when rider weight is added, the postural muscles need to increase their isotonic capabilities to avoid the back hollowing or ventro flexing. In a riderless horse these muscles act to ensure that the necessary rigidity of the main frame is sustained because the back forms the central strut of the body mass. To enable the hind limb thrust to push the body over the planted forelimb, back movement must be reduced to a minimum.

The lateral joints of the equine back also ensure stability. Side bending is not catered for in the anatomical design and the joints between the base of the neck to the junction of the back and pelvis, are not constructed in a way which allows side bending. Neither are there any muscles to achieve a pure side bend. In order to execute such a movement the entire mid section of the equine vertebral column must rotate. This movement is uneconomical for survival in the wild so the postural reflexes of the equine resist the rotational torque continuously, the local muscles working to retain the straight but flexible rod. Circling creates this torque, thereby activating the small anti-torque muscles, improving, over a period of time, their tone, and thus improving the ability of the horse to carry rider weight.

If the neck is left free on a lunge the musculature works as nature intended. If the head is positioned by restraint, the neck musculature has to learn to work to hold the position. The static muscle work necessary for this is very demanding. Head and neck normally enjoy the elastic recoil of the *nuchal ligament* and so muscle activity is minimal for energy conservation (Fig. 9.4). With the head restrained in an abnormal position, this normal elastic recoil is not available for the maintenance of the cervical curve or to prevent the head being pulled downward by gravity. If the neck muscles are forced to support the weight of the head and also resist gravitational pull, the musculature must work in an isometric fashion largely in the inner range. This is extremely tiring and creates muscle fatigue. After a minimum of 3–5 minutes the restraint should be removed and the horse allowed to stretch its neck and to enjoy the elastic recoil of the nuchal ligament once more. This enables the muscles to refuel and recover before the restraint is re-applied.

On a lunge the limb muscles have to learn to balance the body weight over the limbs on the inner side of the circle and to adjust all limb movements to avoid limb collision. The muscles of the hind limb on the outer side of the circle deliver the greatest thrust. They are working concentrically and are required to achieve enough power in the middle range to propel the body mass with little help from the inner hind quarter. These muscles work in their inner range and mainly eccentrically.

To work correctly on a lunge is an excellent gymnastic activity, but no

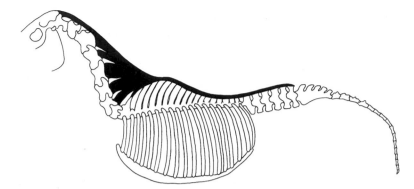

Fig. 9.4 (a) The nachal ligament stretches from poll to withers, continuing to the loins attached to the spines of all the vertebra. In the neck, extensions span the gap from mane to neck vertebra, so the neck vertebra are suspended by the ligament. The stretch on the ligament is determined by the position of the head, and the flexion or curve created by the angles between the vertebrae of the neck. The position of the back is linked to head and neck position.

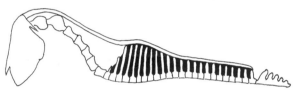

(b) The gentle curve of the neck creates tension from poll to withers, continuing to the loins. The tension lifts the back, enabling the horse to work correctly when carrying rider weight.

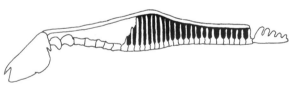

(c) The long and low working position. The lowered head and stretched neck create stretch throughout the nuchal ligament from poll to withers. This stretch continues through the supra spinous ligament (the extension of the nuchal ligament), lifting the back.

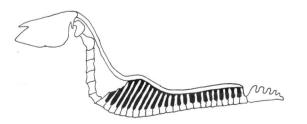

(d) The nuchal ligament is slack due to head position. The area from withers to loins has little support and a 'hollow' has been created in the centre of the back. With the back positioned in this hollow shape hock engagement is impossible.

horse should continue this activity for longer than 15 minutes at a time. It must be allowed recovery periods. As the horse becomes proficient and balanced the inclusion of a line of poles, and later raising the poles to convert them to cavaletti, introduces progressive loading.

The distance between individual poles must be judged by the rider in conjunction with the length of stride of the individual animal. The distances must obviously be constantly adjusted because there will be different requirements at each pace. Animals that have become used to voice command and respond to it well can be loose-schooled, even incorporating poles into the exercises. Jim Grant's 'Rosie', a member of the United States Three Day Team, is a perfect example of this. Jim stands in the middle of an arena with poles arranged at various strategic points and directs Rosie by voice alone.

The following are mistakes made by those unskilled in lungeing:

- To allow the horse to rush
- To allow the horse to lean in
- To allow the horse to work on two tracks
- To allow the horse to choose its own pace
- To imagine that the horse is working as it ambles or runs

If you are unable to lunge correctly or you do not have the facilities, learn to long rein.

Long reining

All the great masters of equitation taught and still teach horses using long reins. There are four schools of long reining. Each requires the use of two reins but the angulation of reins to operator is different in each school. The English method is probably the most practical unless the person working the horse has been trained by a Master of the Classical School.

Long reining is also an excellent way for the trainer to enhance his or her own pre-season fitness campaign!

The tack is identical to that used when lungeing, but two lines 20–25 feet long are required (Fig. 9.5). The horse is tacked up in snaffle bridle, with elasticated side reins running from snaffle ring to the roller on which three or four sets of rings are mounted at varied heights from the girth attachments. A cavesson with three rings on the noseband serves as the anchor point for the reins. The inner rein, attached to the inner cavesson ring passes, in the English method, directly to the trainer's hand. The second is attached to the outer cavesson ring and lies on the far side of the horse to be passed through a chosen ring on the far side of the roller. The rein passes behind the hind quarters under the tail lying 9–12 inches

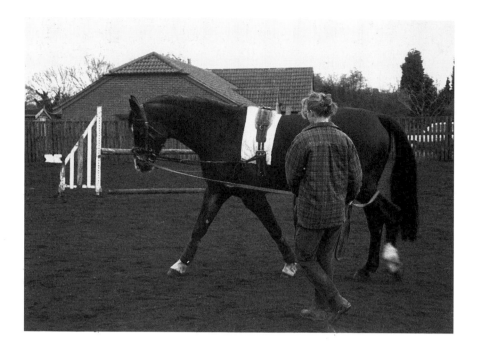

Fig. 9.5 A horse in tack for work in long reins. The horse is wearing: a snaffle bridle with a pair of elastic reins to a roller; a cavesson with three nose rings. The long reins are buckled to the two outer rings and the inside rein passes from nose to the handler. The outside rein passes from the nose, along the outer side of the neck to be threaded through a ring on the roller. It then passed backward under the tail to the handler. The handler walks behind the girth, approximately level with the stifle joint. A horse can be lunged in similar tack, the lunge line being buckled to the centre ring on the cavesson.

above the hocks. The rein continues on to the trainer who should have one rein in each hand. The horse is driven between the two reins, the trainer positioned slightly behind and to the inner side of the hind quarters of the animal. It is important that the reins are neither too slack (Fig. 9.6) nor too tight (Fig. 9.7).

The reins should exert the same pressure as if the animal were being ridden – the inner rein controls direction, the outer assists in the balance of the hind quarters. The horse can be worked on a circle or in straight lines. Changes of direction can be incorporated although this necessitates adjustment of the inside rein which must be threaded through a ring on the inner side of the roller at a height similar to the outer rein. It takes a little more practice to work this way and a novice handler will require help from an expert.

The addition of lateral work will increase the gymnastics of any exercise programme in a manner difficult to achieve by a novice working a horse

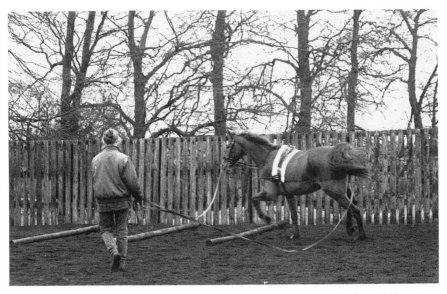

Fig. 9.6   The long reins are too slack, particularly the back rein. This has occurred because the handler has positioned herself too far forward in relation to the horse.

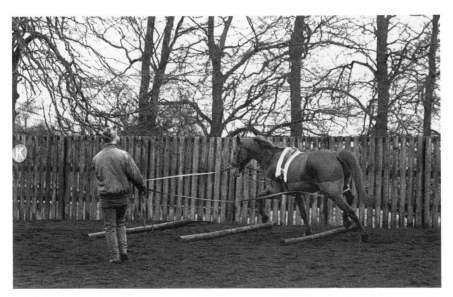

Fig. 9.7   The front rein is too tight, causing the horse to flex its neck inwards towards the handler.

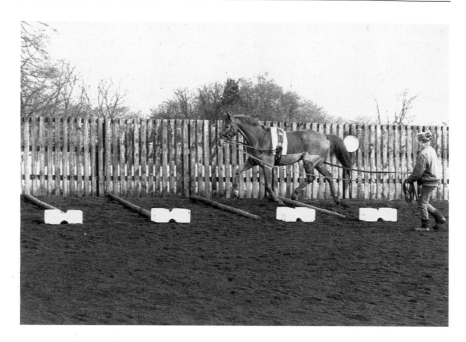

(a) A horse working correctly in long reins down a line of poles. There is no tension on either rein or in the side reins. The horse is working on its own natural outline in a balance appropriate for its conformation.

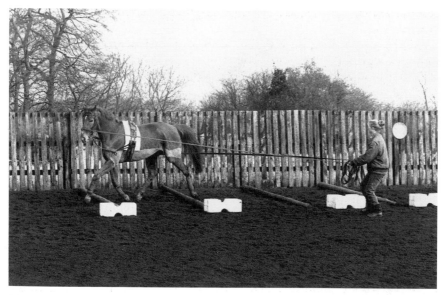

(b) A horse working in an incorrect manner in long reins. This situation has probably been created by the handler who has failed to move sufficiently and is therefore pulling the horse inwards and off balance.

Fig. 9.8

on a lunge. The introduction of poles and cavaletti further increases gymnastic scope (Fig. 9.8a,b) if done correctly. The brilliant muscle building afforded by passage and piaff is also possible to achieve.

Possibly one of the greatest advantages of long reining is the ability to watch the horse work from all angles, allowing for the early detection of problems. All mature horses will benefit from work in long reins, not just those horses who are unbroken to saddle. The method is also extremely useful when trying to encourage a horse to go forward and to take contact with the bit, particularly in animals who have tended to go not only behind the bit but who are no longer achieving the necessary forward propulsion from behind.

Work in hand

To work a horse in hand, the rider or trainer is positioned just behind the horse's head and nearly level with its shoulder (Fig. 9.9). One hand holds the reins just below the bit and the other holds a long dressage whip. This whip is held in the manner of a fencing foil and employed as described by Linda Tellington-Jones in her treatise on wanding. The horse usually wears normal tack, its saddle and a snaffle bridle.

The method is a very valuable aid in training. The horse learns to collect itself round the back, work in balance and, most importantly, engage from behind. Lateral work, square halts and rein backs are also achieved using this method.

Exercises in hand are performed at a walk and at trot, the aim of the trainer working the horse being to achieve gentle restraint by the use of the hand on the reins, at the same time as encouraging forward movement by gentle tapping with the whip. The whip is used either in the exact position where leg aids would be applied or by touching the horse's thigh.

Work in hand is commonly used in Europe but there are few trainers in the UK who employ the technique, although building, balancing and collecting before rider weight is added have enormous advantages. Done correctly over a period of time the performance of horses worked in this manner will improve dramatically.

To summarise gymnastic exercises

- Lungeing is used to teach limb coordination, to build back muscles by the use of the circle, and to selectively load the outer and inner limbs.
- Long reining teaches balance, coordination, change of direction and encourages the horse to go forward.
- Work in hand achieves collection and forward impulsion.

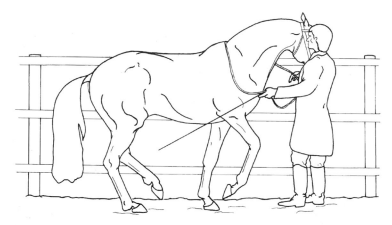

Fig. 9.9 Working a horse in hand. This method is designed to teach collection through the entire body. It takes great skill to work a horse in hand.

The use of poles and cavaletti

Poles

Poles can be used to:

- Vary stride length
- Improve joint proprioception
- Improve muscle coordination
- Re-establish balanced limb activity following injury.

Varying stride length (Figs 9.10–9.16)

Teach the horse to go over one pole at walk and trot before laying out a complicated grid or fan. The distance between poles is always an issue for debate as every horse has a differing stride length and its conformation will determine the length achieved. A horse with a good, sloping shoulder will be capable of a far longer stride than that of a horse with a straight shoulder.

To calculate a distance applicable for an animal, walk it down the long side of a freshly harrowed school and measure the distance between the imprints of fore and hind feet. Do the same at trot. Work out the pole distances from the pattern of hoof prints. Progress from one to two poles then up to four and finally to six, and change the distances between the poles to vary both length of stride and pace. The horse works harder at middle paces than at extended paces when the elastic recoil of tendons and ligaments aids activity.

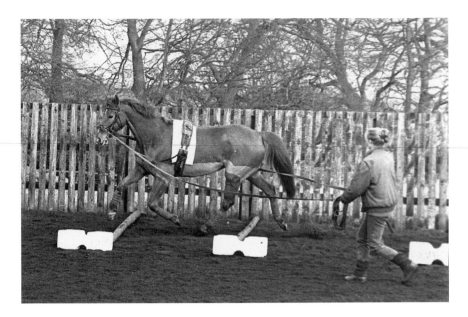

Fig. 9.10   Teaching a horse trot work over poles. The distance between the poles is suitable for this horse – the left hind limb will be put midway between the poles.

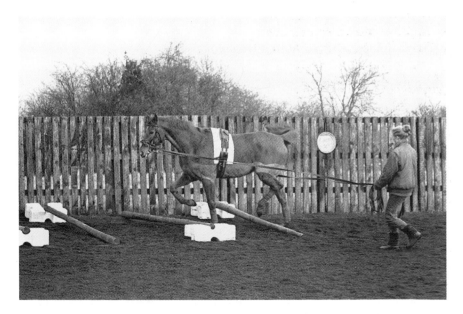

Fig. 9.11   Poles with blocks arranged to shorten the stride at trot. This arrangement of poles achieves increased limb flexion, working the muscles in their middle range.

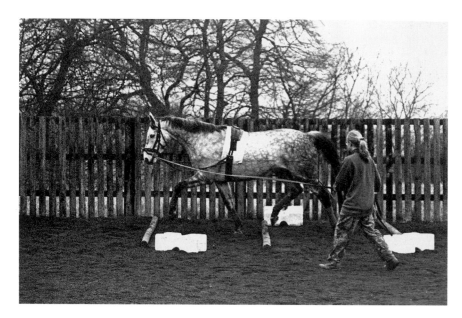

Fig. 9.12   Poles arranged to increase stride length at trot. This arrangement of poles achieves increased limb extension, working muscles in their outer range.

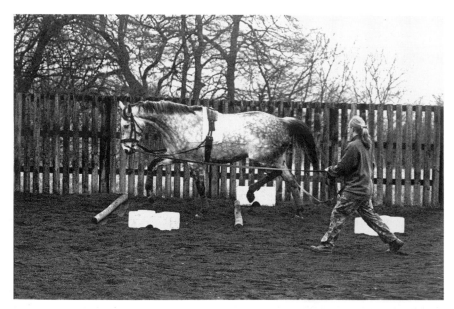

Fig. 9.13   A horse unable to lengthen. The right front foot and left hind foot will put down before passing over the poles. The handler has not moved fast enough and is pulling the horse inward and off balance.

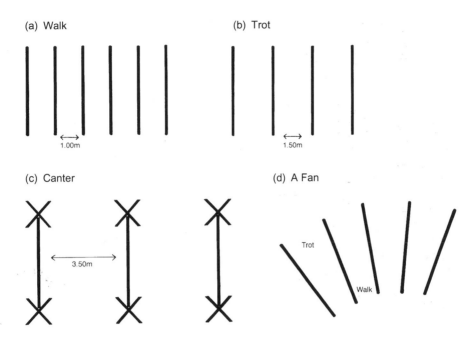

(a) Walk

1.00m

(b) Trot

1.50m

(c) Canter

3.50m

(d) A Fan

Trot

Walk

Fig. 9.14   The use of poles to vary muscle activity. The distances given here are average and must be adjusted for each horse.

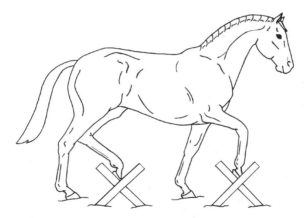

Fig. 9.15   Raised poles achieve muscle activity in the middle to inner range. Stride length can be influenced by alteration of the distance between the poles.

Improving joint proprioception

Joints are loaded with sensors, known as proprioceptors, which communicate with the centres of movement coordination in the brain. The greater the variety of experiences the joints encounter the wider the proprioceptive appreciation. Fans of poles and varied distances, either

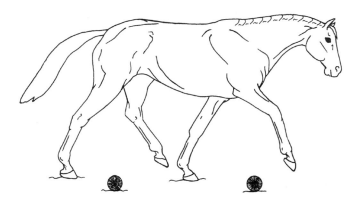

Fig. 9.16 Ground poles achieve muscle activity in the middle to outer range. Stride length can be influenced by alteration of the distance between the poles.

between poles in a line or between poles on opposite sides of the arena are helpful.

Improving muscle coordination

Arrange poles at canter distance down one side of the school and at trot distance down the other. Poles are arranged to be incorporated with the horse working on a circle. Every variation tests coordination as the individual limbs learn to move in differing circumstances to avoid collision with either the poles or each other.

The horse has four limbs to coordinate, and the centres in the brain from where movements are initiated are pre-programmed to avoid at all costs contact between a hind foot and fore leg. This could sever a tendon and for survival in the wild this is catastrophic. Horses do on occasions over reach or clip a fore leg with a hind foot and good coordination, trained by varying the exercises, helps to reduce the risk.

Re-establishing balanced limb activity following injury

A horse that is in pain, even if this is sub-clinical, will alter its movement patterns to avoid that pain. A horse hurting in a front limb will shorten its stride because a series of short strides reduces the weight bearing period of each limb. How often does one hear, 'He used to move like a dream. Now look, no stride at all'?

When the reason for the change in stride has been sought, found and removed, the short stride will remain because it has become the habitual movement. Work over poles, starting with them close together and gradually increasing the distance, will, over a period of time, restore by re-education the original stride pattern. Pole work can be done both from the ground and ridden.

Cavaletti

Cavaletti are poles raised off the ground 6–8 inches. They are either purpose built or are constructed by using two blocks, available from most horse requisite centres, and a pole.

Cavaletti work achieves:

- Coordination (horse and rider)
- Balance (horse and rider)
- Muscle strengthening (horse)
- Discipline of movement (horse and rider)
- Preparation for jumping fences (horse and rider)

As with pole work the horse should start over one cavaletti with a gradual progression until a grid of six or eight is mastered. As with poles, start with a walk and progress to trot and then canter. The horse can be taught from the ground but riding cavaletti is an excellent exercise for both horse and rider.

Coordination

The rider will experience a different 'feel' from each horse at walk, trot and canter. When horse and rider begin to adapt to their individual movement patterns to compliment each other, coordination is beginning to occur.

Balance

The horse imparts a differing feel at each pace due to its balance requirements. Therefore different gait sequences all necessitate varied limb coordinations and balance variation. The rider must adjust to these variations in an imperceptible manner in order to avoid putting the horse further off balance.

Muscle strengthening

Grids progressively load equine muscle as the horse works to lift its legs to clear the poles. The rider will begin to implement and fine tune the closed chain reflexes discussed in Chapter 7 when isometric activity for lower limbs was considered. Rider rhythm is also involved riding down a grid.

Discipline of movement

Work in an arena is contained work requiring a disciplined approach, partly necessitated by the space available but also because the activities are lessons, not just work. Repetition, the spacing between the cavaletti and the number of cavaletti, require control, concentration and effort.

Preparation for jumping fences

To jump fences successfully horse and rider must be in harmony. During the moments leading up to the fence the rider may need to use restraint to ensure the horse meets the jump correctly but at no time should the rider interfere with the horse when it is in the air. To achieve this requires a very big learning curve. Small fences can be constructed using cavaletti enabling the rider to extend their experience before progressing to greater heights and starting to school over fences.

Chapter 10
Progressive Muscle Loading II: The Addition of Skills

In any training regime the long, slow distance work (LSD period) involves both the horse and the rider, the work undertaken aimed at conditioning and improving muscle tone, while, at the same time, the skeletal system of the horse begins its adaptive processes. At the end of this period, six weeks for older horses who have had a short 'holiday', eight to ten weeks for those returning to training after a long lay off, twelve weeks for youngsters starting their career, progressive muscle loading should be increased.

During the LSD period some of the activities listed should be incorporated, interspersed with riding out, both to add variety and to begin to include short lessons. Riders, particularly novice riders, should try to incorporate the exercises 'off horse' as suggested in Chapter 3 during the LSD period. Then, as both horse and rider begin to tone their individual musculature, it is time to join the two together in a series of ridden gymnastic activities. All dancers, no matter what is to be their eventual dance discipline, start with the basic principles laid down by the exercises of the classical ballet school, and no matter what is to be the eventual discipline of the riding horse, thoroughbred racing horses excepted, the fundamental principles of the equine classical school provide an invaluable set of activities.

Nuno Oliveria said 'the horse is not a machine, it is a living being. One rides him and he never forgets the movements he has learned, but what the rider must remember is it is necessary to know and to always give the commands correctly. Always return to basic exercises and spend time with them'. The rider should be so sensitive that he can feel from the back of the horse and should know even if the horse has slept in a bad position in his stable. The tactful rider feels if part of the horse is tired and knows how to engage this part and to change the forces to other areas. Oliveria also states that 'all riders must try to relax their hands and have a light contact'. In order to achieve light contact a rider must have a seat independent of their hands.

As described earlier in the text, ridden work over cavaletti is an excellent way of improving rider balance and also an excellent way of increasing the loading for the horse, particularly if the animal has previously been worked over cavaletti from the ground. A useful learning and improvement routine for both horse and rider is to work a horse in the arena with the cavaletti poles arranged down one long side at walk spacing and on the other long side at trot spacing.

All activity should begin with the horse ridden on a loose rein around the arena, then gradually achieving more collection. When the animal is warmed up and the rider begins to relax in the saddle, the horse is ridden down the line of walk placed cavaletti, circles, and is ridden down the trot placed cavaletti. Both these activities should, if possible, occur on a loose rein in order that the horse must balance itself and become accustomed to carrying rider weight as it varies limb movements to step over the raised poles. Cavaletti work should not be continued for longer than a maximum of 15 minutes. At the conclusion of concentrated lessons the horse could be taken out for its normal long slow hack.

As both rider and horse become more confident over the lines of poles the distances can be adjusted in order to either lengthen or shorten stride and small fences introduced at the end of a line of poles.

It really does not matter if the horse is new to training or an older horse returning to training. As Oliveria said *always return to the basics at the beginning*.

Cavaletti not only progressively load muscles but also improve suppleness and balance, as well as initiating the closed chain reflexes necessary for both horse and rider to jump fences. When horse and rider have learned to balance down a line of cavaletti at walk, trot, both extended and collected and at canter, due to the fact that lateral and medial stability of all the limbs is extremely important, some of the basic classical movements need to be incorporated. These do not need to be performed to the level required at Grand Prix dressage. Some of the exercises were designed to train the muscles concerned with limb stability, others to achieve collection. Because the movements required are small, cadence is also improved. Cadence might be described as rhythm combined with energy. As cadence begins to improve so the horse will be able to move softly from one type of movement to another, an imperceptible, smooth transition.

Of the basic classical exercises the two which are of the most use for the general purpose animal are the *shoulder in* and the *half pass*.

Shoulder in

The most successful way to teach a horse a *shoulder in* is to ride a perfect geometric circle of approximately 10 metres at walk, continue circling two or three times and then, as the arc of the circle meets the long side of the school and the horse begins to bend, to try to continue the circle by applying the appropriate aid (inside leg just behind the girth, release, close). The horse will come off the circle and continue down the side of the school. A similar shoulder in exercise is shown in Fig. 10.1.

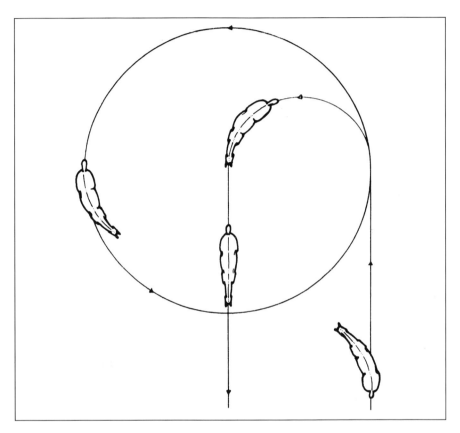

Fig. 10.1   A trained horse performing a shoulder in and improving discipline by returning to a straight line down the centre of the school.

An important rider requirement is to remain in balance over the centre of the horse and not to lean in to the circle.

Serpentine

As the horse learns the commands and begins to execute the shoulder in comfortably, it is possible to progress to a serpentine (Fig. 10.2).

It is an excellent suppling exercise and creates concentric work for the

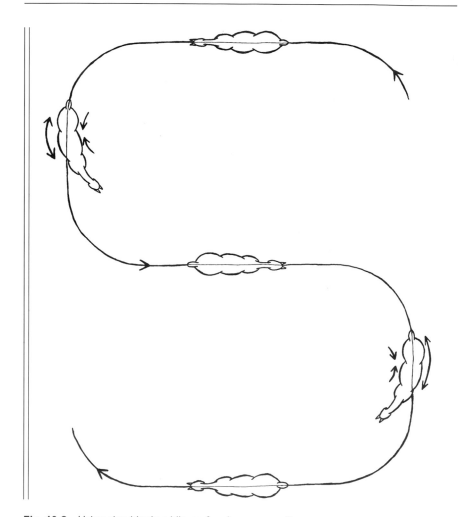

Fig. 10.2 Using shoulder in while performing a serpentine.

adductors and abductors of both of the forelimbs and both hind limbs in a manner that is impossible to achieve on a straight line.

Half pass

When the horse has mastered the shoulder in and learned to move away from the leg it is time to begin to teach the half pass (Fig. 10.3).

Start with a shoulder in, asking for this at the middle of the long side. Continue as far as the middle of the short side, then turn down the centre line still in the position of shoulder in. Then apply the outside leg lightly, pushing the horse sideways in the position of a half pass for *two or three steps only*, then relax and allow the animal to walk straight.

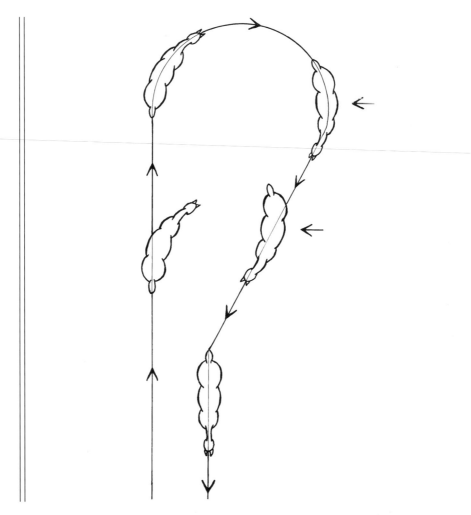

Fig. 10.3 Learning the half pass. Begin as for a shoulder in but continue off the circle. A preparation for suppling exercises.

Once both rider and horse are comfortable at both shoulder in and half pass they can be executed at trot. Both are excellent suppling exercises and both load and activate the muscles of adduction and abduction of all four limbs in a manner impossible to achieve when riding a circle or straight line (Fig. 10.4).

Due to the slight lateral position of the neck adopted, particularly during shoulder in, the muscles at the base of the neck are exercised. They are not visible but lie adjacent to the bones at the junction of neck to chest (thoracic cage). These muscles are very important in all horses as

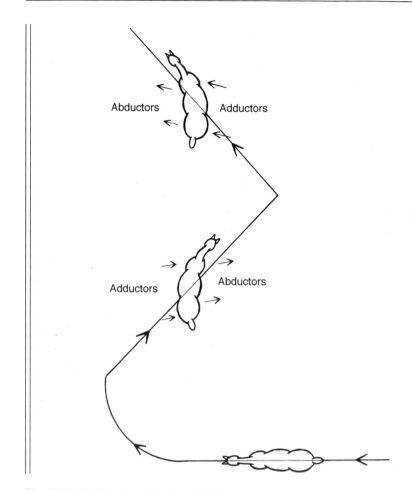

Fig. 10.4 Working the adductor and abductor muscles using a half pass.

stabilisers for the first rib. Jumping ability is seriously impaired if these muscles are not developed.

If the horse has been performing all the varied activities relatively readily and then, one day, seems unwilling to work, do not persist. Take the animal out for a ride and try again another day. It may be that you, the rider, are not concentrating and are giving incorrect commands, or the horse may have become thoroughly bored and for some reason is not going to make any effort.

When giving lessons (to the horse) the golden rule is *to practise in walk and get it right before progressing to trot*, not only because you are trying to imprint a closed chain reflex, but also because the effort required both mentally and physically will be greater at trot than at walk.

The progressive loading of the musculature continues by introducing canter to the horse's programme both in and out of the school. Progression from walk to canter achieves balance and suppleness. Start by changing from collected trot to canter, then down to collected trot, before attempting walk to canter. When the attempt to change from walk to canter is made, make certain that the horse is on a circle then, when on the circle and in a corner, apply the aids for canter. It is essential that the horse learns to move into a canter smoothly.

Progressive loading, ridden work over cavaletti and simple classical exercises should all continue to be included in general training until the suppleness and obedience required for the eventual task have been achieved. The length of time it will take for this to occur will vary with each horse dependent on its early training, its muscle capability, its learning ability and its attitude. There is a reason for going back to the basics even with an old horse, because the horse, while it may have learned some of the movements required, has to learn a set of slightly new commands from each rider. It is extremely difficult for a horse to be trained and schooled by one person and then ridden by another. Great riders are in tune with their horses and able to ride apparently any horse without previous experience of the animal. Notables today in the United Kingdom would be Frankie Dettori and John Reid, flat race jockeys, Graham Bradley and Jamie Osborne, National Hunt jump jockeys, Blyth Tait and Mark Todd, three day eventing, Carl Hester, dressage, and possibly the just retired David Broome from the show jumping fraternity.

Adequate exposure to competition requirements

No matter what the eventual level of excellence or competition requirement, pre-competition exposure to all expected demands is essential, not only for success but also to avoid injury as far as possible by pre-conditioning tissues.

For example, horses trained for endurance in flat areas that suddenly meet the heather covered slopes of Exmoor are rather like skiers who have never experienced powder snow, confused and off balance. It is therefore sensible for the rider and trainer to have understood fully, by attending events before competing, the requirements of that competition.

One of the more difficult things for a horse to do is to jump downhill, when a considerable amount of eccentric work is demanded. Muscles and tendons can learn what is expected in this situation but only after gradual exposure to the activity (Fig. 10.5). If you wish to teach your horse to jump downhill, start over small obstacles on easy inclines and gradually increase the size of the fence. Then find an incline with a steeper angle and

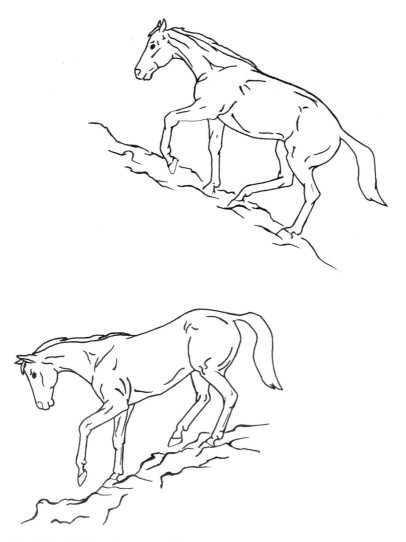

Fig. 10.5 Uphill work – concentric and progressive muscle activity. Downhill work – very demanding eccentric muscle activity.

use the same procedure, small fence first then gradually make the task more difficult.

Do not attempt any new activity more than four or five times at each session – muscles and all soft tissues tire easily when exposed to new tasks.

Many of the training areas attached to French racing centres are sited in wooded areas. There are countless trails through the woods, themselves on hills. Nearly all the tracks have fences of differing types and heights, allowing riders to trot, canter and gallop their animals over a variety of obstacles. Fences are also sited on uphill and downhill slopes. Jumps into water are another hazard necessitating a huge learning curve and require practice. Have you ever jumped into water and tried to run? It is often possible with the cooperation of local landowners, to create similar training conditions to those enjoyed in France.

Once basic learning has been experienced and balance and coordination trained, the patterns become a cortical imprint. No experience will ever mirror competition exactly, but remember, few outdoor competitions (be they endurance, showing, jumping or event) take place on manicured, flat surfaces such as are found in the 'all weather' arena or on the 'all weather' track. There is little point in preparing in perfect conditions then having to compete on a rough, probably undulating or sloping surface. Wild horses or animals turned out on moors, bogs, hills or mountains, are all far more balanced than those living in flat, level conditions. *As sure footed as a mountain pony* is very pertinent.

Appendix 1
Programme Design

Many people, especially those newly introduced to horses, find it incomprehensible that there are no definite, written down recipes for training. Training is an art. If you understand the effects of the varied activities called exercises, you should be able, as a rider or trainer, to select a combination best suited to the individual requirements of the animal in question.

First considerations

Horse	Age
	Conformation
	Previous experience
	Current level of fitness
	Previous problems
Rider	Expectations
	Experience (training, riding expertise)
	Time available
	Own fitness
Facilities	School or arena
	Gymnastic apparatus (poles, fences)
	Local hacking facilities
Discipline	Levels of competition aimed for
	Spacing between competitions
	Specialist requirements

When planning a training programme it is essential to understand the difference between *work* and *lessons*.

Work

Work develops the horse's strength, improves cardio-vascular efficiency and prepares the animal for lessons.

Lessons

Lessons involve obedience, that is a gradual learning by the horse to respond and perform to rider command and, by so doing, execute the movements or perform the activities required by the rider.

Lessons follow work, the work having settled the horse before asking for concentration and full attention. The time allocated for each individual lesson should be short. The horse has a small attention span and endless repetition 'to try to get it right' will cause fatigue, boredom and even resentment, dependent upon the individual temperament of the animal.

It is advisable, if the horse keeps making mistakes, fails to learn or perfect a new activity, to change the lesson, returning to try again later. The rider or trainer should reflect on their input: were the commands clear? Was the horse correctly balanced? Who went wrong – horse or trainer? To give muddled signals makes it difficult for the horse to respond correctly. In a way it is like a person trying to understand the instructions for setting a new watch if those instructions are in Russian and the purchaser can only read English.

Lessons should be interspersed throughout the *work* programme. The following points are useful when considering designing a programme:

- Work from the ground in long reins and on a lunge are excellent for both correction of faults and the building of postural and activity muscle groups.
- Periods of long, slow distance work must be incorporated into the final work programme following its use in early preparation.
- Riding out across fields, over commons or park land, in woods, across moorland, in hill or mountain country keeps both horse and rider alert and entertained, improves balance in both, improves coordination between rider and horse, and improves reflex responses in all the joints of both.

Vary the activities when on a ride. If there is an even stretch with a useful hedge, practise, for example, a shoulder in, change pace, incorporate variety. In Sweden this type of riding is used with great success. Training has tended to become very stereotyped and far too regulated. Lighten it. Even if you do not incorporate scientific interval training within the general programme, by monitoring the heart rate and its return to normal you will have a good indication of the level of fitness achieved.

When you are satisfied that the horse is ready to compete start with small local events, preferably those that will mimic the eventual demands of your discipline. For example endurance riders might consider taking part in a sponsored 10 mile ride, horses could jump at clear round events at local riding clubs, event horses could take part in hunter trials, dressage horses and event horses could compete at small, non-taxing competitions. Make these experiences pleasant and mentally stressless for your horse by not asking too much of it. Make these outings a self learning curve, no need to panic if a vital girth has been left behind. It will not happen a second time and it is better to make mistakes when it is not an important event rather than at the first serious competition, for a disciplined approach is as essential for the rider as it is for the horse.

Artificial training aids

There are a variety of training aids. All undoubtedly have a use, but unfortunately they may be incorporated into training at a very early stage, usually before the horse has been worked sufficiently to build an adequate musculature. This musculature when conditioned may enable it to achieve the position naturally, without the need for the aid.

Many problems associated with the position of the head, neck and back are created rather than cured by the inappropriate use of an aid. The modern conception of an 'aid' seems to be that they are designed for changing the position of the horse's head and neck in an endeavour to put the horse into what is assumed to be a correct outline. Just as it is quite impossible to achieve exactly the same seat position in a group of riders, so it is impossible to achieve an exact outline in a variety of differing horses. The use of the various reins undoubtedly affects the position of head and neck, but they should never be used by a person who does not have effective legs, for the fore and hind ends of a horse must move in a synchronised fashion. Without effective legs it is impossible to ensure that hind quarter activity mirrors that of the forelimbs dictated by the use of the various reins or aids.

To work on the forehand only, without correct engagement of hock and hind quarter muscle is a waste of valuable time. The horse will learn to go in a manner which achieves collection and activity in front, due to the enforced change of head and neck position, but with no impulsion from behind.

Running rein

William Cavendish, Duke of Newcastle (1592–1676) designed the running rein (Fig. A.1). It was commonly used throughout the period of classical

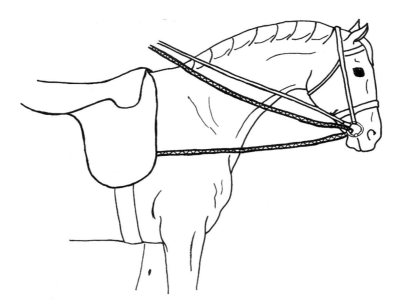

Fig. A.1 The running rein.

education. The rein was fastened under the saddle flaps before returning via the bit rings to the rider's hands. The rein passed from the inside to the outside of the bit ring and was similar to a draw rein. There is, however, a difference in the action of the two. The running rein causes the nose to be brought inward but places less emphasis on the lowering of the head, allowing the horse to balance its back in a manner to which it has become accustomed and is comfortable. The purpose of this rein is to increase the isometric toning activity of the muscles of the neck.

Draw rein

The draw rein (Fig. A.2), as its name suggests, draws the head downward as well as causing the nose to be brought in towards the chest. The idea of the rein is to assist in shortening and to achieve a rounded outline. The rein is fastened to the girth and, like the running rein, passes from the inner side of the bit ring to the outer and thence to the rider's hands.

The running rein is rarely used today but the draw rein has become common, as people attempt to create an outline in many cases before the horse's musculature has been sufficiently prepared to achieve the required shape. One of the main problems with the draw occurs because horses ridden in them continuously tend to become used to them, leaning upon the restraint of the rein in order to balance.

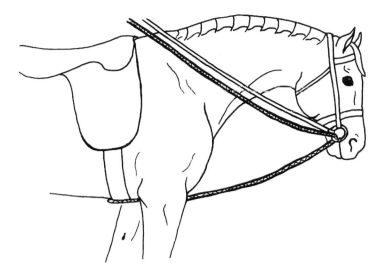

Fig. A.2 The draw rein. The discerning rider should decide during progressive training if the horse needs to both lower the head and flex, in which case the draw rein would be the rein of choice. If flexion only is required the running rein would be preferable.

Many horses also tend, with overuse, to go behind the bit. As forward progression is one of the most important attributes of the well-trained horse, this is not helpful.

The balancing rein

This type of restraint was perfected by the late Major Peter Abbot Davis. It was vigorously promoted in the press and through public demonstrations given throughout the United Kingdom. The object of the balancing rein was to try to build the muscles of both back and neck in a relatively short space of time.

There are three ways of fitting the Abbot Davis balancing rein. First, there is a straight attachment from mouth to girth, the second from tail to mouth, and the third from the mouth upward. The design incorporates rubber sections which work as springs, with the angles of the straps employed acting as pulleys. It is a system that necessitates instruction from an expert to achieve success.

It is interesting to note that the use of a rein attached from the tail to the mouth can be seen in the carvings of the facade of the temple of Ramesses the III when chariot horses were tail reined to counter both one sidedness and a lack of impulsion from behind. The principle behind the Abbot Davis is that the back is rounded and the quarters are actively brought under the body at the same time as the head and neck are lowered. The idea appears, once again, to be an attempted short cut in order to produce the outline.

The Chambon

The Chambon (Fig. A.3) was designed to re-school animals who had adopted an unnaturally high head carriage and developed an upside down neck and was designed to be used on the lunge. Invented in France the rein is rarely used in the UK although it is common in many European training establishments, and is the subject of a book published in 1988 by J.A. Allen.

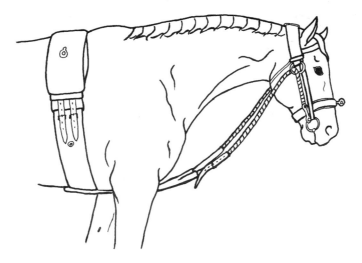

Fig. A.3   The Chambon is used to teach the horse to lower the head and neck so as to raise the back of the animal. Raising the back closes the scapulae (shoulder blades), allowing freedom of forelimb movement, in turn ensuring hock engagement.

The girth of saddle or roller acts as an anchorage for the strap which passes upward and splits, looking rather like an elongated running martingale. Each strap continues to the poll where each is threaded through a ring sited just below each ear and attached to either end of a padded cavesson headpiece. Each strap then passes downward, parallel with the bridle cheekpieces, to be attached to the ring of a snaffle bit.

The device, useful as it is, has little or no 'give' as has the latest rein based on similar principles.

The bungee rein

This is constructed from a single, strong rubber cord, shaped as an elongated 'U', the centre of which is passed through a moveable constrictor to afford length adjustment (Fig. A.4). The centre of the 'U' and adjustment clip is placed at the poll. The two arms are passed down on either side of the cheek straps, through the snaffle rings and continue downward to meet at the girth, where each clips to a centrally placed noose through which the girths have been passed. Adjustment for length is achieved by moving the constrictor ring on the cords at the poll. The rein is very kind, encouraging flexion throughout the neck complex, so achieving the back lift necessary to allow hind quarter engagement.

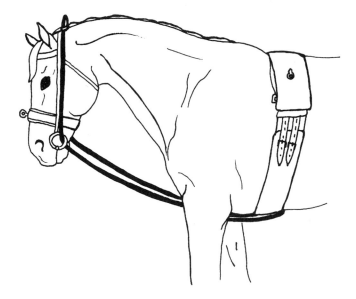

Fig. A.4   The bungee rein. This is the newest training aid and can be used both when working the horse from the ground and when riding. It is a useful 'reminder' when reschooling animals.

The De Gogue

This rein was also developed in France. The De Gogue (Fig. A.5) was designed to be used by experts to correct, when riding, problems at the poll, base of the neck in a horse described as 'strong'.

The cords which in the Chambon are attached to the bit, pass through the snaffle rings to continue as a rein, allowing considerably more rider influence. The device, as with all other aids, was developed for use by experts rather than novice riders. Although originally conceived to correct problems, a theory suggested that its usage also built the muscles of the adopted position and that once those muscles had developed, the position would be retained automatically.

(a)

(b)

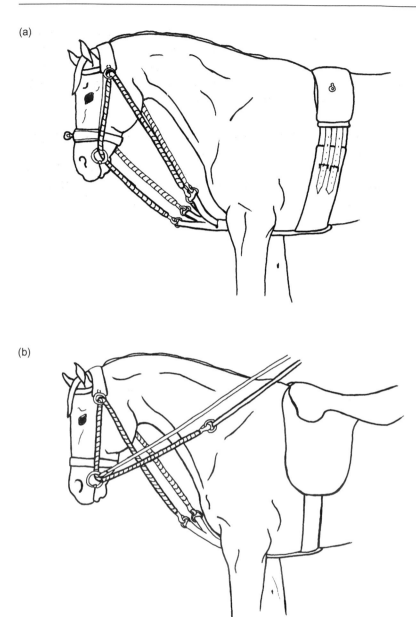

Fig. A.5 The De Gogue can be used for both lunge and ridden work. The aims of early training are to teach the horse to raise its back using the unique construction of the neck, interacting as it does with the support of the back.

The reins described here are methods of increasing the resistance to the activity of muscle, thereby improving their competence, but the methodology employed by the reins does not imprint a brain response that will be automatically generated once the reins have been removed. This is because the horse needs the command, given by the rein, in order to activate the response.

If a horse is not going forward as it should, or is not adopting the positions required by the rider for its particular discipline, it is far better to go back to the beginning and start once again in long reins before resorting to highly sophisticated training aids, each one designed by a 'master' of equitation. The bungee is probably the only exception.

Appendix II
Man versus Horse

The studies available show that the horse, in athletic terms, is superior to man. The physiological changes resultant from heavy exercise have been assessed in both species and demonstrate the following differences:

- Muscle tissue accounts for 41% of body mass in the horse, 45% in man.
- Respiratory exchange in the horse under exercise conditions is nearly twice that of man.
- The cardiac output in the horse under exercise conditions and calculated per kg of body weight is twice that of man.
- During exercise the concentration of circulating haemoglobin in the horse doubles. There is a scarcely perceptible increase in man.

These findings show that the interaction between the spleen, heart and muscles in the horse is more efficient than in man due to:

(1) A higher concentration of arterial oxygen.
(2) A greater cardiac output.
(3) A more efficient extraction of oxygen during activity.

Although subject to similar 'waste' during activity, the horse appears able to:

(1) Tolerate higher blood lactate levels than man.
(2) Still maintain a lower blood pH than man.
(3) Tolerate the increased acidosis.
(4) Demonstrate a greater capacity to buffer (resist) acid/alkali changes in the blood and tissues than man.

A feature common to both appears to be that both species demonstrate inadequate lung function. In the horse this may be caused by rider weight and the effects of the girth.

The horse demonstrates a physiological activity superior to man but an inability to achieve its potential *possibly* due to impaired respiratory ability. Only a few physiological variations have been isolated by research, but there would appear to be sufficient evidence to suggest that concepts associated with human athletic performance may well not be pertinent to the horse. Man, for example, has a preconceived idea of his body's requirements, both during training and at competition. Man decides, before running a marathon, what he will eat the previous day, how long he needs to warm up – he has the ability to *decide* his course of actions, he has a brain allowing him to think and plan ahead. Not only must the horse do exactly what it is commanded by the rider but it has *no idea* when taken to a competition, for example, how long the journey will be, what lies in store at the other end, the tasks it will be expected to undertake. There is no way a horse can preconceive and prepare. Man prepares mentally, but how can the horse do so? There are two species to train – the art is to prepare both, then bring them together to perform as a team.

Appendix III
Health Maintenance in the New Age Horse

Keep the top door of the loose box open at all times and increase the number of rugs to maintain warmth. Make certain there is adequate air-flow through the stable, but not cold draughts.

Shavings for bedding

Damp slightly if dusty or change your supplier. Sweep walls and ledges regularly while the horse is out of the box to remove any residual dust.

Paper bedding

Print dust is a chemical hazard arising from poor quality newsprint. If you find a fine grey black dust on walls or ledges you have a chemical dust problem. Damp or change the bedding.

Straw bedding

Avoid dusty, short straw. Shake up the bed with the horse out of the box.

Rugs

Shake daily outside the box away from the horse.

Grooming

Groom in a well ventilated area, outside if possible. Why pollute the horse's box with its dust, leaving particles suspended in the air for the animal to inhale, or for you to inhale while you are grooming?

Hay

Shake up hay in a well ventilated area and shake again just before feeding. Dust shaken out of the hay will sink back on to it if the hay is beneath its own dust cloud. Always check for mould. *Do not use mouldy hay or haylidge type fodder that is fermenting.*

Disinfectants

Remember that all disinfectants, just like chemical sprays, must kill in order to be effective. That is their purpose, to destroy harmful life forms to ensure that the local environment is rendered inhospitable for the pathogens to reproduce. The sprays and disinfectants are designed to lose their toxicity after a period of stated time. Do not ignore the time periods stated. If you spray a box wearing a mask and then put a horse into the area before the spray has detoxified the horse will inhale the toxin.

Chemical sprays

Avoid riding through any area that has recently been sprayed, particularly if it has not rained since spraying commenced. Avoid any area where aerial spraying is in process. Avoid any area where sheep have been dipped. The National Farmers Union have at last accepted the fact that all dips are dangerous. If spraying your own land or yard, read and follow the instructions. They are printed for very good reasons – all chemicals are highly toxic.

Indoor arenas

All indoor arenas should have a sprinkler system. If dust is seen on any surface, it has come from somewhere. It may have been thrown into the air by horses working on the surface. Eventually, like snow, it settles. If dust is there to settle it is there, in the air, to inhale. Increase the ventilation and damp the surface to prevent the dust from getting into the air.

All weather surfaces

There is a kick back of fine particles at speed no matter what the manufacturers claim. On all weather gallops jockeys wear goggles to protect their eyes, but the horses are inhaling the dust the jockeys are avoiding. All weather surfaces *must* be maintained to the standards advocated by the manufacturers as this will reduce the likelihood of particle inhalation. However, it *will not* totally remove it.

Travelling horses

Horse boxes and trailers should be well ventilated, remember that as a moving vehicle cuts through the air deflecting it sideways a vacuum is created at its rear. Suction then pulls air into the box from behind the transport. This air is usually chemically polluted by exhaust fumes. Horses lucky enough to be near an open window press their noses to the gap trying to breathe fresh air from outside the box. Remember that, while travelling, the horse is working to balance for the entire journey and muscle work requires oxygen. Four horses in a lorry use a lot of air and expel an awful lot of waste. Leardon (Irish Equine Research) has shown most horses travel in chemically polluted air and that the levels of pollution enhance the ability of various bacteria and microorganisms to reproduce, reaching problematic levels in a very short time.

Man is free to both choose and change his environment: if a room is stuffy he can open a window. The domestic horse is forced to endure conditions created by man: he cannot control the ventilation of his stable or of his transport. A great deal of lung damage occurs as a result of thoughtlessness on the part of the horse carer. Remember, the lungs of both man and equine are very delicate and they need consideration and care.

Epilogue
The Fundamentals of Putting Sports Science to Work

There are no short cuts to fitness and no therapies or aids which are going to improve an animal's capabilities. Just as trained athletes, all horses have a level of capability. This level may be constrained by several features, and the first is conformation. Some horses are quite unable to perform certain tasks because their conformation does not allow them to do so. The second is mental attitude: horses that have been mentally damaged at some time in their career (they may have suffered a considerable amount of pain, or have become bored and dissatisfied) will be very very difficult to change. These sort of animals need a total change of venue and training programme.

Always bear in mind that:

- Horses' bodies adapt when exposed to small, regular increases in exercise (progressive loading).
- Unless progressive loading is achieved, the response to training will be negligible.
- Any increase, too fast or too strenuous, can produce unwanted results including tissue damage.
- Muscles respond quite rapidly to loading and exercise but structures such as bone, ligaments, tendons, joints and the feet take time.
- You are not training one single structure, you are training a complicated interaction of systems.
- Never neglect the endurance type of long, slow, building work.
- The speed of an activity and the distance that the horse must cover are two separate entities.
- As the training programme develops, develop speed independent of distance.
- Physical and physiological effects are not instant and the result of training will not show for three or four days after an increase in work. A horse may respond to a sharp bout of interval training on the day in question, but three days later be dull and unable to perform simple tasks, this indicates progression has been rushed.

Remember that response to training slows with ageing. Never forget that each horse, just like each person, is also an individual and will respond in a slightly different manner from others in your stable.

It is of course perfectly possible to ride a horse from the field or from the stable without any attempt at improving its physical fitness, and many horses do survive in this manner. However if you wish to compete, to enjoy your horse and for your horse to enjoy you, it is sensible to build in some form of athletic training programme. Europe has done this for years. The British tended to regard the Classical School and European teachings as 'foppish' because to them riding was not an art. The horse was a means of transport, an agricultural necessity. For pleasure, it was used for racing. No one built riding schools as they did in Europe.

Today's scientific knowledge and the inclusion of scientific principles into training has apparently allowed horsemen to achieve ever increasing feats of excellence with their mounts. However, when we consider the conquests by Alexander the Great, even Napoleon, it is as well to pause and to wonder if today's feats really are a first, or if the horse after World War I just took a back seat, making way for the early excitement created by the motor car, and if we are merely, as the twentieth century draws to a close, rediscovering its amazing versatility.

Useful Addresses

The Alexander Technique
Maxine Shenton, MSTAT, BHSAL Church End Cottage, Great Hormead, Buntingford, Hertfordshire SG9 0NH
Tel: 01763 289235

Rideaway Style & Fitness Horse
Richard Perham   Game Cottage, Earls Court Farm, Lambourn Woodlands, Hungerford, Berkshire RG17 7SB
Tel: 01488 73963
Mobile: 0836 521636
Fax: 01488 71433

Hilton Herbs Ltd
Downclose Farm, Downclose Lane, North Perrott, Crewkerne, Somerset TA18 7SH
Tel: 01460 78300
Fax: 01460 78302
e-mail: hilton.herbs.ltd@dial.pipex.com

Natural Animal Feeds Ltd
Penrhos, Raglan, Monmouthshire HP5 2DJ
Tel: 01600 780256
Fax: 01600 780536

The Laminitis Clinic
Robert Eustace MRCVS
Wooton Bassett
Wiltshire

Index

Note: subjects applying to the **rider** are clearly marked, all other subjects apply to the **horse**.